Mental Health Care in Paramedic Practice

Ursula Rolfe and David Partlow

Printing history
The authors and publisher welcome feedback from the users of this book.

Please contact the publisher:

Class Professional Publishing,
The Exchange, Express Park, Bristol Road, Bridgwater TA6 4RR
Telephone: 01278 472 800
Email: post@class.co.uk
Website: www.classprofessional.co.uk

Class Professional Publishing is an imprint of Class Publishing Ltd

A CIP catalogue record for this book is available from the British Library

Paperback ISBN: 9781859599242

eBook ISBN: 9781859599235

Cover design by Hybert Design Ltd, UK
Cover image courtesy of South West Ambulance Service NHS Foundation Trust
Designed and typeset by Newgen Publishing UK
Printed in the UK by Short Run Press

This book is printed on paper from responsible sources. Refer to local recycling guidance on disposal of this book.

Contents

About the Authors

Dr Ursula Rolfe is a principal academic and deputy head of the Midwifery and Health Sciences Department at Bournemouth University. Within this role, she is also Practice Simulation Lead for the Health Sciences Faculty. Ursula has a PhD with the focus on how paramedics manage patients experiencing mental health from the University of Southampton and has presented her work at various national and international conferences. She has been the national Mental Health Lead for the College of Paramedics since 2014 and continues to support and initiate change for frontline paramedics within this arena and feels it is vital to highlight the need for further education, training and support. This book was the next step in terms of identifying means to support her fellow paramedics in managing mental health patients. She continues to publish and initiate research within this field while maintaining her clinical practice as a paramedic prescriber in urgent care.

David Partlow is currently a Strategic Manager within Adult Social Care in Somerset. David joined the NHS in 1996 after six years in the Army, serving in the Royal Electrical and Mechanical Engineers. David progressed through operational management within the ambulance service and subsequently spent 11 years as a Clinical Development Manager and Senior Clinical Lead. Amongst other things, David was the Mental Health Lead at his trust and represented them at the National Ambulance Service Mental Health Group. He has undertaken sessional lectures on the Mental Capacity Act and Mental Health Act at universities in the South West region and has represented the ambulance service on the National Steering Group for the Crisis Care Concordat and the independent review of the Mental Health Act. Moving into Adult Social Care, David is responsible for in-patient mental health, social care, the AMHP service and adult safeguarding. Since the onset of the COVID pandemic, David has also been the COVID-19 lead for Adult Social Care, responsible for providing guidance and support to the care sector. Outside of work, David is the Vice Chair and Trustee of a suicide bereavement charity and coaches and helps run the minis and juniors section of his local rugby club.

Chapter contributors

Will Murcott is a Mental Health Nurse and Senior Lecturer at the Open University. Will is passionate about inter-professional working and the importance of mental health care across all disciplines in health and social care. Will has a strong clinical interest in pre-hospital mental health care, having worked in many community settings with children, young people and their families. Will's career has been across many different settings including secure services and CAMHS inpatient and community care. In his educational capacity Will has supported paramedic pre-registration training, providing teaching on mental health care and the legal aspects to mental health care. He has contributed to the JRCALC Clinical Guidelines and his research areas of interest are young people's mental health.

Carol Robertson is an Advanced Clinical Practitioner and Paramedic. She recently began working at East Cheshire NHS Trust within the Older Persons' Assessment & Liaison (OPAL) team following a long career with the North West Ambulance Service. Her roles included Community Specialist Paramedic, Specialist in Telephone Triage and Paramedic Supervisor. Carol developed her interest in older adults during her time working within telephone triage where she recognised there was a high volume of calls relating to older adults who had fallen. As she progressed to the role of Community Specialist Paramedic she developed her skills, knowledge and interest in delirium, frailty and ageing. She graduated with an MSc in Advance Clinical Practice in 2020. Within her Trust she developed eLearning modules for all clinicians and non-clinicians on the topic of delirium and (alongside colleagues) developed a frailty eLearning module for all staff. In addition to this, she has delivered a podcast for the College of Paramedics on Older Adults plus two CPD webinars. Within her Community Specialist Paramedic role Carol has delivered falls and frailty awareness to ambulance clinicians, independent living communities, older persons groups such as lunch clubs, WI and U3A. She has also developed a falls and frailty training presentation for care and nursing home staff. At home Carol is married to a fellow paramedic and their lives revolve around their dogs!

Aimee Yarrington has been a qualified midwife since 2003. She has worked in all areas of midwifery practice, from the high-risk consultant-led units to the low-risk stand-alone midwife-led units. She left full-time midwifery practice to join the ambulance service, starting as an Emergency Care Assistant and working her way up to Paramedic while always keeping her midwifery practice up to date. She has worked in several areas within the ambulance service including the emergency operations centre and the education and training department. Her work towards improving the education of pre-hospital maternity care has led to her receiving a fellowship award from the College of Paramedics. She strives to improve the teaching and education for clinicians in dealing with pre-hospital maternity care.

Case study contributors

Huw Corness	Paramedic and Lecturer in Simulation
Stephen Down	Mental Health Lead
Melissa Doyle	Lecturer (Paramedic)
James Field	Student Paramedic
Andrew Hichisson	Advanced Paramedic Practitioner (Urgent Care)
Justin Honey-Jones	Paramedic, Urgent Care Practitioner and Associate Lecturer in Paramedic Science
Tom Mallinson	Prehospital Care Doctor, Rural GP and Paramedic

Melinda (Dolly)
McPherson   Advanced Clinical Practitioner (Paramedic)
Jo Mildenhall   Mental Health Project Lead
Sarah-Jane Niles   Paramedic

The case studies in this book are real cases provided by practising clinicians. The content follows particular assessment frameworks, including the Mental State Examination (MSE); (see M. Soltan and J. Girguis, How to approach the mental state examination, *British Medical Journal*, May 2017). The case studies represent the clinician's recollection of events. We accept that recall bias may impact some of these recollections.

Preface

The original Institute of Health and Care Development paramedic course equipped, in just 12 weeks, the ambulance technician with the knowledge and skills required to manage the vast range of clinical scenarios which paramedics face. At least that was the proposition. Within that 12-week course, the mental health component was brief at best and provided what can only be described as a cursory overview of the law as it stood at that time. No focus was given to describing a mental disorder and no time was set aside to support the paramedic in developing the skills needed to support those in crisis.

Just as the world has moved towards a greater awareness of mental health and wellbeing, so too, has the paramedic profession. There is, though, a long road ahead and still much to do to truly deliver the parity of esteem needed between physical and mental health. One cannot be separated from the other and both are intrinsically linked. Greater awareness and acknowledgement are needed of the vital role that paramedics play in supporting those in crisis and greater investment is needed in developing the educational foundation that will enable paramedics to effectively support and deliver the clinical interventions required.

We, the authors, have a passion for mental health, for the paramedic profession and its role in supporting those in crisis. We hope that this book will provide insight and generate debate regarding the standing of mental health within the ambulance service and also the wider remit of the paramedic profession. We truly believe that the paramedic profession has a great deal to offer a developing and further integrated health and social care system. We hope that this book will support paramedics to better understand mental ill-health and the fundamental statutory provisions associated with mental health and mental capacity, and also encourage a growing desire to see mental health as a core part of paramedic clinical practice.

Introduction

Ursula Rolfe and David Partlow

Introduction to themes and context of mental health for paramedics

The ambulance service has changed a great deal over the last 20 years. Demand has grown exponentially and the range of observations, assessments and interventions has expanded way beyond what many of us in the ambulance service could ever have envisaged. The rise in activity and demand on ambulance resources has not been limited to physical health needs and has increasingly seen ambulance crews being dispatched to support people in crises related to their mental health.

In 2019, 168,000 mental health calls were made to London Ambulance Service, its staff attended over 105,000 incidents where the originating complaint related to mental ill-health. This equates to roughly 8.9% of total incidents the service attended in that year and is in most likelihood an underestimate of the true volume (London Ambulance Service, 2020). Marsh (2017) likewise suggested that information obtained through a Freedom of Information request identified that the number of ambulance activations for 'people experiencing mental health problems in England' had increased by almost 25% in the preceding two years. Paramedics had been dispatched to over 30,000 more patients who had made contact describing a mental health crisis in 2016–17 (172,799) compared with 140,137 in 2014–15. However, accurate data on mental health calls is complex and not easy to obtain. Triage systems used within ambulance control rooms attempt to identify the chief complaint and record this as a single clinical call reason. Data which is based on such triage systems therefore relies on the information provided by the caller being an accurate reflection of the clinical need.

Reflecting on the Institute of Health and Care Development (IHCD) Paramedic Award that preceded the move to higher education, mental health education was restricted to an appreciation of the law as it pertains to the Mental Health Act 1983 and in particular Sections 2, 3, 4, 135, and 136. This equipped the paramedic with a rudimentary knowledge of those sections at best and did not provide an awareness or understanding of the various presentations that the newly qualified paramedic would be required to attend.

Has this changed with the move to higher education provision and awards? A rudimentary review of the prospectus and module content of many universities would raise the question of how far educational provision has improved with respect to mental health and many readers may wish to reflect on their own experiences.

Paramedics often report frustrations when dealing with incidents related to mental health crisis. A lack of education in this regard promotes a feeling of insufficiency which leaves paramedics feeling uncomfortable and unable to fully meet the needs of the individual in crisis (Rolfe et al., 2020).

Yet, despite issues with a lack of detailed educational and pre-registration exposure to the management of mental health crisis, we have a clearly defined vision whereby the management of mental health crisis should be viewed in parity with the management of physical health crisis and within that an expectation that all healthcare providers will rise to meet that challenge.

The Crisis Care Concordat

In February 2014, organisations with a significant interest in supporting those in crisis came together to commit themselves to the principles of The Crisis Care Concordat. The Crisis Care Concordat, fundamentally sought to further the cause of those suffering from mental health crisis and to address the significant disparity and lack of equity between the provision of care to those whose crisis derived from a primary physical health issue compared to those with a primary mental health issue (HM Government and Mind, 2014).

The Concordat required individuals responsible for policing, health, housing, primary and secondary care, social care and charitable provision to come together to remove organisational boundaries and to look at how a collaborative approach could improve access to services and outcomes for individuals. This created an opportunity for all organisations to engage in a conversation that sparked debate and developed a greater awareness of the importance of mental health that has in no small part created the demand for change that we have witnessed ever since.

Why it is important

The National Institute for Health and Care Excellence (NICE), the government body that provides national advice and guidance to improve health and social care, acknowledges that individuals who experience poor mental health are equally more likely to experience poor physical health, and that individuals with enduring mental ill-health will, on average, die 10–17 years earlier than the national average (NICE, 2019). Poor mental health is often linked to chronic physical illness. Naylor, et al. (2012) suggest that this is true in 46% of cases. The Mental Health Foundation (2021a) suggests that individuals with the highest rates of self-rated distress are more likely to die from cancer and that individuals diagnosed with schizophrenia experience double the risk of death from heart disease. They are also three times more likely to die of respiratory disease.

Is poor mental health driving poor physical health or is poor physical health driving poor mental health? Where does social deprivation sit within this and how can it be addressed?

It is not possible to separate physical and mental health from the wider debate regarding the health of the nation, both must be addressed equally. Reducing health inequalities and promoting physical and mental wellbeing are essential components of a healthy population.

This is a complex area where it is not always easy to describe cause and effect; however, we know that individuals with poor mental health are far less likely to be in receipt of physical healthcare and are less likely to be in receipt of support regarding healthy eating and smoking and alcohol cessation (Nursing, Midwifery and Allied Health Professions Policy Unit, 2016).

The Percy Commission, recommended in its 1957 report that the provision of care should be moved from an institutional basis to community provision (Grounds, 2001). In many instances, over 60 years later, that transition is still happening. While the physical separation of those suffering from mental ill-health is changing, there remains a significant lack of understanding and a very high degree of stigma and shame associated with mental ill-health.

The responding paramedic is often the first point of contact for an individual in crisis, that initial response is crucial in reassuring the individual that we care, that their crisis has been acknowledged and that we are ready and able to provide that initial support (NHS at 70, 2019). It is vital that we do not contribute to the disparity of esteem and that the paramedic profession acknowledges the role it plays in supporting all those in crisis.

Additional vulnerabilities

Charles et al. (2019) define population health as being a mechanism by which a focus on improving physical and mental health and wellbeing is undertaken alongside a drive to reduce health inequalities which often drive poor outcomes. This holistic approach is required if we are to tackle the root cause of physical and mental ill-health. Providing employment opportunities, improved housing options, access to education and social enrichment are all vital if we are to resolve the root causes of ill-health in the population.

There are very clear links between mental ill-health in children and adolescents and the prevalence of health and social care inequalities (Mental Health Foundation, 2020). Children and young people in the poorest households are three times more likely to have a mental health problem than their more affluent neighbours.

Evidence suggests that 50% of mental health problems are established by the age of 14 years and 75% by the age of 24 years (Murphy and Fonagy, 2012). This was supported by Hagell and Shah (2019) who stated that 75% of mental health problems start before the early 20s and that 14.4% of 11–16-year-olds and 16.9% of 17–19-year-olds in England met the criteria for having a mental disorder at the time of the 2017 Mental Health of Children and Young People survey. Therefore, fundamentally, if we do not address the additional vulnerabilities that exist within childhood and especially where children experience social deprivation, we have already failed and, thus, the current focus on raising the profile of mental wellbeing and encouraging people of all ages to talk about how they feel becomes ever more important.

The NHS Long Term Plan

In early 2019, the NHS Long Term Plan was published. This document set out the key objectives for the NHS and how services would be delivered over the next 10 years (Charles et al., 2019). The long-term plan reinforces the commitment to deliver the Five Year Forward View for mental health and to create greater access to and availability of services to support those in crisis. This will include the provision of single points of access or services with 'no wrong door' principles. There is a growing momentum and a genuine commitment behind calls to improve mental health services for the future. Investment in mental health services will have increased by £2.3 billion by 2023/2024 (NHS, 2019).

Importantly, given the significant underinvestment in children's and adolescent mental health, there is a significant emphasis on the development of effective services for children and young people (NHS, 2020).

Structure of the book and overriding themes

Throughout this book we will attempt to raise the debate of mental health within the context of paramedic practice from the frontline and 999 perspective, as well as additional case studies from a wide variety of paramedic experiences which include primary care. We will look to provide an awareness of inter-professional considerations and where the ambulance service and the paramedic profession fit in the health and social care context.

We will look at the complex nature of decision making with respect to mental ill-health and suicidal ideation and raise the importance of open communication with respect to the analysis of risk.

We will then consider the most prevalent mental health conditions paramedics are exposed to in practice. Each condition will have an illustrative case study written by paramedic colleagues from across the UK. We will provide an overview of the mental health condition as well as its management, according to national guidelines. For paramedics, the case studies should be read in conjunction with local clinical guidelines and protocols depending on the area of practice and should not replace clinical judgement. For paramedics and other readers, we also hope to dispel some of the myths associated with specific disorders. This book will also look at special considerations associated with mental ill-health.

Throughout this book we have been very conscious of the terminology associated with mental health. The Mental Health Foundation (2021b) provide a useful guide to terminology for further reference. In this way we hope to be part of the continued movement to reduce the stigma associated with mental health which still exists.

Finally, we will look to the future and what role the ambulance service and paramedic profession may have in respect of mental health and how to manage presentations of mental ill-health.

It is hoped that this book will prompt reflection, debate and support for paramedics so that we are better equipped to respond to the challenges that lie ahead for all of us.

References

Charles A., Ewbank L., McKenna H. and Lillie W. (2019). The NHS long-term plan explained. *The King's Fund*. Available at: https://www.kingsfund.org.uk/publications/nhs-long-term-plan-explained#mentalhealth

Grounds A. (2001). Reforming the Mental Health Act. *The British Journal of Psychiatry*, 179(5): 387–389.

Hagell A. and Shah R. (2019). Key Data on Young People 2019. London: Association for Young People's Health.

HM Government and Mind (2014). About the Crisis Care Concordat. *Crisis Care Concordat Mental Health*. Available at: https://www.crisiscareconcordat.org.uk/about/

London Ambulance Service (2020). Episode 6 of 'Ambulance' highlights the growing pressure on ambulance staff responding to mental health patients. Available at: https://www.londonambulance.nhs.uk/2020/10/21/episode-6-of-ambulance-highlights-the-growing-pressure-on-ambulance-staff-responding-to-mental-health-patients/

Marsh S. (2017). Ambulance call-outs for mental health patients in England soar by 23%. *The Guardian*. Available at: https://www.theguardian.com/society/2017/aug/13/ambulance-call-outs-mental-health-patients-soar-23-per-cent

Mental Health Foundation (2020). Mental health statistics: children and young people. Available at: https://www.mentalhealth.org.uk/statistics/mental-health-statistics-children-and-young-people

Mental Health Foundation (2021a). Physical health and mental health. Available at: https://www.mentalhealth.org.uk/a-to-z/p/physical-health-and-mental-health

Mental Health Foundation (2021b). Terminology. Available at: https://www.mentalhealth.org.uk/a-to-z/t/terminology

Murphy M. and Fonagy P. (2012). Mental health problems in children and young people. Annual Report of the Chief Medical Officer 2012, Our Children Deserve Better: Prevention Pays. Available at: https://assets.publishing.service.gov.uk/government/uploads/system/uploads/attachment_data/file/252660/33571_2901304_CMO_Chapter_10.pdf

NHS (2019). NHS Mental Health Implementation Plan 2019/20–2023/24. Available at: https://www.longtermplan.nhs.uk/wp-content/uploads/2019/07/nhs-mental-health-implementation-plan-2019-20-2023-24.pdf

NHS (2020). Next Steps on the Five Year Forward View, Chapter 5: Mental health. Available at: https://www.england.nhs.uk/five-year-forward-view/next-steps-on-the-nhs-five-year-forward-view/mental-health/

NHS at 70 (2019). Mental Health in the NHS: Changes and experiences. Available at: https://www.nhs70.org.uk/story/mental-health-nhs-changes-and-experiences

National Institute for Health and Care Excellence (2019). NICEimpact mental health. Available at: https://www.nice.org.uk/media/default/about/what-we-do/into-practice/measuring-uptake/niceimpact-mental-health.pdf

Naylor C. et al. (2012). Long-term conditions and mental health: the cost of co-morbidities. The King's Fund and Centre for Mental Health. Available at: https://www.kingsfund.org.uk/sites/default/files/field/field_publication_file/long-term-conditions-mental-health-cost-comorbidities-naylor-feb12.pdf

Nursing, Midwifery and Allied Health Professions Policy Unit (2016). Improving the physical health of people with mental health problems: Actions for mental health nurses. Available at: https://assets.publishing.service.gov.uk/government/uploads/system/uploads/attachment_data/file/532253/JRA_Physical_Health_revised.pdf

Rolfe U., Pope C. and Crouch R. (2020). Paramedic performance when managing patients experiencing mental health issues – Exploring paramedics' Presentation of Self. *International Emergency Nursing*, 49: 100828.

Part 1

Mental Health in the Context of Paramedic Practice

Chapter 1

Interprofessional Considerations

David Partlow

Introduction

No one organisation is responsible for supporting those with mental health needs. This is often a complex and collaborative area of health and social care practice. In this section we will look at the roles played by a number of partners in providing clinical care and support to individuals with mental health needs.

There are, as in any area of healthcare, different opinions about the role organisations play within mental health and, in particular, how that role could, or should, develop in the future. In many respects the role of organisations relating to mental health has developed over time and has done so organically in response to the developing demand; as such it has not been taken forward in a planned or coordinated way. This has led to a huge variance across the country in terms of how individual organisations respond to those in crisis.

General practitioners

Often the initial point of contact for health services, General Practitioners (GPs) are called upon to provide an initial assessment for a myriad of physical and mental health concerns. Therefore, the role of primary care in the assessment, initial management and treatment of mental health problems is a crucial one.

England (2020) for the Royal College of General Practice (RCGP), suggests that one in six adults and one in ten children are likely to have a mental health problem in any year and that 90% of people with mental health problems receive the totality of care within a primary care setting. Further, the RCGP goes on to suggest that approximately 30% of people who make appointments with their GP will have a mental health aspect to their illness. Given the significant relationship between physical and mental health perhaps this is unsurprising, but it does indicate the significance of managing patients' needs in a holistic manner, taking into account both physical and mental health aspects.

GPs will, in consultation with specialist services, manage the daily needs of those accessing mental health services and often act as a gateway to secondary services for further specialist intervention.

There are a number of developing models where primary care is engaging in innovative practice, for example, the co-location of mental health professionals within GP practices. This provides an opportunity to intervene earlier in supporting the mental health needs of the community and to provide a more seamless transition into secondary services, if required. Through the development of a more holistic approach primary care is better placed to enable improvements in both physical and mental health.

The NHS has also acknowledged that the provision of psychological therapies within primary care supports earlier intervention; utilising a therapeutic approach to improve both physical and mental health outcomes may help to reduce future burden on health services (NHS, 2021).

It is further acknowledged by NHS England that the early availability of mental health therapy in primary care is particularly useful in terms of the provision of targeted therapy for older adults with common presentations such as anxiety or depression (NHS, 2021).

The role of allied health professionals is developing in the growing multidisciplinary primary care workforce. Indeed, many paramedics now work as part of that team; it is therefore a natural extension of this that we incorporate mental health professionals within that extended primary healthcare team.

Police

Police colleagues are often the first responders on scene when calls are received to respond to those in crisis. Similar to paramedics, education in mental health has not kept pace with the changing requirements of operational work and as such, police officers are often faced with situations and scenarios that they are not best placed to manage.

While police have powers under the Mental Health Act (2007), all such powers have limitations and police officers are often ill-prepared to manage situations for which they have received little training or preparation. The report, 'Policing and Mental Health: Picking Up the Pieces', suggests that it is untenable that people experiencing a mental health crisis are provided with a response from police officers rather than a response from an appropriate healthcare professional. This same report also concluded that officers are not provided with the support needed and that they do not have the necessary skills to support those in crisis (HMICFRS, 2018).

This aligns with the objectives of the aforementioned Crisis Care Concordat to ensure appropriate health intervention is provided and that the criminalisation of mental health is addressed through reduced need for police intervention. The Force Management Statement issued by the Metropolitan Police (2019) states that it receives a call about a mental health concern once every four minutes and that it responds to a mental health-related call every 12 minutes. This goes some way in describing the demand that mental health calls place on the police service and why many are now trying to better manage that demand to reduce the impact on the wider service.

Police forces are now looking to reduce the demand caused by the current need to transport individuals to hospital because an ambulance is not available, and where delay would be unsafe for both police and patient. They are seeking more appropriate ways of supporting people in mental health crisis, such as that received from those who are clinically trained. They are looking to reduce time spent in emergency departments providing a degree of security while assessments are undertaken or appropriate health facilities found. Many forces are increasingly reluctant to provide what are often described as 'welfare checks' on vulnerable people unless evidence of harm is provided. This is a significant problem and places additional demand on their workload; it may not always be the best use of their time given rising rates of crime in many areas.

However, the debate regarding police involvement in mental health crisis is not solely about demand management, it is a fundamental conversation about whether it is appropriate to dispatch professionals, whose focus is on the provision of law and order to support those who have committed no unlawful act or transgression.

Police officers have powers to detain an individual under Section 136 of the Mental Health Act and to support the removal of that individual to a place of safety. This can be undertaken if the police officer has reason to believe that the individual appears to be suffering from a mental disorder, they are not currently in a private dwelling (a house, flat or room where that person is living, this includes a private garden and garage), and they are in need of immediate care and control. Since the Policing and Crime Act (2017), police must make every effort to consult a registered medical practitioner, a registered nurse, approved mental health professional (AMHP), occupational therapist (OT) or paramedic prior to utilising the powers. It is interesting to note that paramedics are included within the group of consulting health professionals. This may suggest a growing realisation that mental health crises are the responsibility of health services therefore the role of the paramedic and the ambulance services in the treatment of such patients should be expanded.

On balance, police officers have a broad responsibility to protect the public and promote safety in the community and as such, they have a role in supporting those in crisis. However, if we are to truly provide a parity of esteem between physical and mental health (a phrase promoted within the Crisis Care Concordat to express the desire to see physical and mental health on an equal footing), we need to work together to reduce the stigma and decriminalise police involvement in mental health crisis. The Independent Commission on Mental Health and Policing report (Adebowale, 2013) makes it clear that the police will always be required to attend incidents where individuals may be presenting with mental health difficulties. However, the report also makes clear that police resources should not be used in isolation as the primary response as such needs are best met through health and social care intervention.

The College of Policing's report 'Authorised Professional Practice' (2016) discusses the common misconception that individuals in mental health crisis pose risk to others. The reality is that the greatest risk is to the individual in crisis themselves. Individuals suffering from psychosis are portrayed in various media as violent and aggressive and yet they are far more likely to be victims of crime (Pettitt et al., 2013). The police do, therefore, have a role in protecting individuals from harm and discriminatory behaviour, but that does not mean that they alone should hold that responsibility.

Social workers

The British Association of Social Workers (BASW, 2014) highlights the crucial role played by social workers in delivering outcomes for members of the community with mental health needs. Social workers promote recovery and assist individuals in living independent and productive lives. In essence, social services employees often act as advocates for the human rights of the individual, speaking up for those who cannot be heard.

It is interesting to note that healthcare often focuses on what is wrong with an individual, on providing a diagnosis and subsequently recommending a specific intervention. The approach of social workers, however, is based on recognising an individual's strengths and how they can be supported in achieving personalised goals. It is the social worker who will look at the wider determinants of ill health, housing, employment, gainful activity, social inclusion and social justice.

Varying models of service delivery exist within health and social care; but what is vital when supporting individuals is that both health and social care are engaged and working together to support the individual in their recovery. It is impossible to consider the health and social determinants of ill health as separate entities.

Social workers working in mental health will also require a comprehensive understanding of the complex legal frameworks within which they need to work. This includes reference to the Mental Health Act (1983), the Mental Capacity Act (2005) and the Care Act (2014).

They will specifically be engaged in decision making regarding deprivation of liberty, the application of best interest decisions and in ensuring that the rights of the individual are protected and central to any decisions made for them. Section 117 of the Mental Health Act (1983) places a joint responsibility on health and social care to provide after-care for those detained under Section 3 to prevent re-admission. Health and social care professionals must therefore work closely together to ensure that appropriate care and support is provided to meet the ongoing needs of those who remain eligible through this provision.

Social workers are increasingly working to support individuals within the community, liaising with care providers to develop innovative solutions. Innovations, such as using assistive technology to maximise independence, are helping to reduce the levels of deprivation previously seen within institutionalised care. With this comes the ability to effectively manage risk and to engage collaboratively to enable support where it is required based on the needs and desires of the individuals and their support systems.

Approved Mental Health Professionals (AMHPs)

Following an amendment to the Mental Health Act in 2007, the role of the Approved Mental Health Professional (AMHP) was created. It replaced what was previously known as the approved social worker. The rationale for the change was in part to open up the role to other professions outside social work. Despite this, and the option for mental health nurses, occupational therapists and registered psychologists to undertake training and qualification, the vast majority of AMHPs in most areas are still social workers.

The statutory responsibility for the provision of AMHPs sits with the local authority; however multiple models of provision exist. These range from the provision of 24/7 AMHP services managed and operated from within the local authority, provision of day-time AMHP services within the authority and out-of-hours services managed by a mental health provider trust, to services that are completely managed by a mental health provider trust. There are merits to each different model and many are based on the locally determined need and level of activity.

The AMHP is the health and social care professional responsible for the coordination of Mental Health Act assessments. This is an important point to note, for while it is the responsibility of medical professionals to make appropriate recommendations, it is the fundamental role of the AMHP to decide whether a person should be detained under the Mental Health Act while taking recommendations into account.

This is a really important point: those who are liable for detention should not simply be deprived of their liberty if lesser restrictive options exist. It is also important to consider the wider social determinants of ill health and whether alternative mechanisms or interventions can bring about the same outcome without the need to detain an individual against their will. An example of this would be an individual who has experienced a significant deterioration in behaviours associated with dementia, for example, an increase in violence, aggression or difficult behaviours. Can that individual be managed in a way that supports them and prevents or mitigates the risks they pose to themselves and others while doing so in the least restrictive manner? This is the fundamental role of the AMHP: to consider the relevant legislation and work in accordance with the law, but also, in many respects, to act as the advocate for the individual being assessed; to balance medical recommendations against the rights and needs of the individual.

When undertaking a Mental Health Act assessment, the AMHP must make an application to a named hospital. A recommendation cannot be fulfilled if the named hospital does not have an available bed. This again is important in terms of the timeliness of subsequent transfer to hospital; a significant delay may mean beds are no longer available and the application process will need to be restarted.

The 'nearest relative' is a special term used in the Mental Health Act (1983) which gives one family member certain rights and responsibilities. The nearest relative is not the same as the next of kin, who does not have any rights under the Mental Health Act. If detention in hospital under Sections 2, 3, 4, or 27 of the Mental Health Act is under consideration, the AMHP must make reasonable efforts to identify and contact the nearest relative so that their opinions are taken into account. The nearest relative is not necessarily the nearest living relative in a literal sense and indeed, may not be a relative at all. Nearest relatives can be displaced by a court and might instead be an appointed individual within a statutory organisation such as the local authority.

Should the AMHP make an application for detention, they are then responsible for organising the transfer of the detained person to hospital. This is, for some paramedics, a contentious issue, but perhaps one that may speak to societal and/or paramedics' cultural perception of mental health and an indication of our wider views about the role of the ambulance service. Department of Health and Concordat signatories created the Mental Health Crisis Concordat which called on society to deliver a parity of esteem. This requires anyone detained under the Mental Health Act to be conveyed to hospital in a safe, dignified and timely manner. Police resources should not be used to convey patients unless they pose a risk to themselves or others; in such circumstances, police conveyance may then become the most appropriate mechanism (HM Government and Mind, 2014). That is not to say that the ambulance service should not consider alternative resources, many are now considering the skill set of individual ambulance crew members and the type of vehicle best suited for mental ill-health transfers.

There are a number of misconceptions regarding the requirement for the AMHP to travel with the ambulance crew following any decision to detain under Mental Health Act. The AMHP is responsible for the organisation of the transfer and may attend the hospital in order to provide a handover to nursing staff who then officially receive the application on behalf of the hospital managers. AMHPs may, however, delegate their authority to ambulance crews should they be willing to accept the authority to transport the individual to the place at which they are to be detained. It is therefore not necessary for the AMHP to travel with the ambulance and patient into the ward.

Community Mental Health Teams (CMHTs)

Community Mental Health Teams or CMHTs are multidisciplinary teams working in the community. Team members will come from a number of health and social care backgrounds and include psychiatrists, psychologists, community psychiatric nurses, social workers and occupational therapists. CMHTs will also have links with primary care and others, including third sector organisations.

CMHTs provide support for those where initial support, perhaps from within primary care, has not met the individual's needs or it is felt that support from additional specialists is required. In most cases, referral to a CMHT is managed via the individual's GP.

An initial assessment from one or more members of the team will determine what level of support or intervention is required and this will be managed alongside continued physical health management from within primary care. A number of areas are now developing enhanced services within primary care to enable earlier intervention from mental health specialists which aims to reduce the delays in the introduction of specialist services thus reducing the complexity of handover between services (Rethink Mental Illness, 2021a).

Crisis teams

Crisis teams or Crisis Resolution and Home Treatment (CRHT) teams provide support for those in crisis outside of the hospital environment. Again, the model varies depending on locally commissioned services. For paramedics, there is often a misunderstanding that crisis services can provide an emergency response. In some instances the nomenclature of 'teams' has been introduced to replace 'crisis intervention' in an attempt to better manage expectations of crisis teams' abilites to instantly respond.

Crisis teams are multidisciplinary, working to support and, if possible, de-escalate an individual's developing crisis to prevent admission to an inpatient unit (Mind, 2018; Rethink Mental Illness, 2021b).

Psychiatric liaison

In order to meet the mental health needs of those seeking help from acute hospitals, psychiatric liaison services provide the essential link between emergency departments and inpatient wards. This recognises both the significant demand for mental health expertise within the acute setting and also the correlation between mental health and physical health (NICE, 2018; RCPsych, 2020).

It is worth noting at this point that the NHS Five Year Forward View for Mental Health (Mental Health Taskforce, 2016) has recommended that by 2020/21 all acute hospitals should have an all-age mental health liaison service providing support to both emergency departments and inpatient wards.

Criminal justice

The Centre for Mental Health (2016) suggest that up to 90% of individuals within the criminal justice system have some form of mental health problem or substance misuse problem. This is clearly a concern and an issue that needs to be addressed. The Centre for Mental Health further concluded that while services do exist within custodial establishments, they are often underfunded and unable to effectively meet the needs of the incarcerated population.

Many areas now operate Liaison and Diversion services who seek to identify individuals entering the criminal justice system who may have a mental health issue, a learning disability, substance misuse problem or other vulnerability. The service will then seek to provide support for individuals as they move through the criminal justice system. They will refer into various health and/or social care services to divert them into more appropriate services and away from the courts (Together for Mental Wellbeing, 2021).

Liaison and Diversion services work to identify those at risk earlier within the criminal justice process, prevent the all-too-often seen cycle of offending and improve outcomes for individuals thus reducing the burden placed on the criminal justice system (Rethink Mental Illness, 2021c).

Drug and alcohol services

There is a strong link between mental health services and drug and alcohol services (Jarvis, 2019). In many areas services are closely linked with third sector organisations. They provide brief interventions, therapeutic interventions, support and practical help such as needle exchange. Services will differ based on local needs and commissioning intentions. For more information, see Chapter 15, Drugs and Alcohol and the Impact on Mental Health (p. 185).

Child and Adolescent Mental Health Services (CAMHS)

Child and Adolescent Mental Health Services (CAMHS) provide specialist support to young people who may be experiencing poor mental health. This will include low mood and depression, anxiety, poor self-esteem, self-harm, eating disorders and a range of other problems.

Specialist interventions may be provided to support the individual as with adult services and will include a range of therapeutic interventions, provision of medication or more intensive support. In most areas CAMHS will provide support up until the individual is 18 years old, although this may be extended if appropriate (Mind, 2019).

Third sector engagement

Third sector voluntary organisations have a significant role in supporting mental health services and they are a source of expert advice and lived experience. They conduct research, raise awareness, promote mental health and mental wellbeing awareness and training. This sector also provides direct support to patients and often offers directly commissioned services for individuals.

Individuals suffering poor mental health often gain significant benefit when they are engaged with peers who have similar experiences. Many 'crisis cafes' and other informal service provision for those seeking support prior to crisis are supported or run directly by third sector organisations.

In addition, many suicide bereavement services are provided by third sector organisations. These vital services specialise in the particular and unique needs of those bereaved through suicide.

For any paramedic wishing to know more about mental ill-health, a review of the information held by charities such as the Mental Health Foundation, Samaritans, Mind, Rethink Mental Illness, Heads Together, Papyrus, and many more is a crucial first step.

The Mental Health Act 2007

Many of us will talk about an individual being 'sectioned' and use this phrase without truly understanding what this means for the individual. The Human Rights Act (1998) Articles 5 and 8 outline our very basic human right to freedom and liberty of person and our right to live our lives in a way determined by our own volition. The impact of removal of those rights cannot be underestimated.

Any detention under the Mental Health Act (2007) must always be considered the least restrictive option, based on medical recommendations and supported by law. Detention should not be undertaken lightly, nor should it be the first consideration when determination of support for an individual is being undertaken.

Various sections of the Mental Health Act (1983) are applicable to paramedic practice. Section 135 refers to the powers bestowed on a police officer to detain a person within their own home where they are suspected to be suffering from a mental health disorder and are unable to care for themselves (or are being neglected by others, e.g. carers) to be legally detained in their home and then removed to a place of safety to be assessed under the Mental Health Act (2007). The warrant also allows a patient, who is already detained under the Mental Health Act (2007), but has left a hospital without permission, to be searched for by a police officer and returned to the hospital.

The individual detained under Section 135 can then be kept at the place of safety for up to 24 hours. This can be extended for a further 12 hours, but only if the individual could not, for clinical reasons, be assessed within the initial 24 hours. The period of detention cannot be extended for operational issues, for example, the lack of available beds or staff. The period of detention commences upon arrival at the place of safety or, alternatively, upon arrival of the police if onward transfer does not occur.

The police, in conjunction with the AMHP, will have obtained a warrant from a magistrate which provides lawful means of entry and removal of the individual to a place of safety. The AMHP will have outlined that they have reasonable cause to believe that the individual has a mental disorder and is at risk of harm (Table 1.1).

Table 1.1 The professionals involved and their role.

Job title	Role in relation to Section 135 warrant
Approved Mental Health Professional (AMHP)	An AMHP applies for a warrant if they are satisfied that the patient meets the specified legal criteria. AMHPs work 24 hours a day and every social services department has an emergency team. If the warrant is granted, an AMHP will assess the patient's mental health with an approved doctor.
Justice of the Peace (magistrate)	An AMHP will apply to a magistrates' court for the warrant and will present the evidence they have under oath. A magistrate will hear the application in a closed court or at home. If the magistrate is satisfied that the legal criteria is met, a warrant will be issued. A warrant can be applied for 24 hours a day.
Police officer	If the warrant is granted, it authorises a police officer to be accompanied by an AMHP and a doctor to attend the patient's address and remove them to a place of safety. The warrant grants a police officer the power to force entry if required. If the patient is already detained under the Mental Health Act and absconds, the police officer(s) may attend on their own.
Paramedic/ambulance clinician	A paramedic/ambulance clinician may be requested by the AMHP and/or police officer to convey the patient to a designated place of safety. The clinician may also initiate an AMHP by making a referral if they feel the patient is suffering from a mental health disorder and is not able to self-care in their own home. This would be appropriate if the Mental Capacity Act does not apply, e.g. no life-threatening emergency but the patient is in need of care, however does not consent to conveyance to the emergency department. The clinician could also discuss their concerns with the patient's GP who can also refer to an AMHP if appropriate. A clinician's assessment and consideration of the patient's social circumstances could be useful information for the AMHP to make a decision.

A place of safety

The warrant will specify that the patient must be taken to a place of safety. This can include (patient specific):

- An emergency department
- A mental health hospital
- A police station (only as a last resort or if the patient is a high risk and never for anyone under 18 years of age)
- Residential accommodation provided by social services
- The patient's own home (if they consent)
- The home of a patient's relative or someone they know (if they consent).

There are various myths surrounding the Section 135 warrant. Some are explored and dispelled in Table 1.2.

Table 1.2 Myths and facts about the Section 135 warrant.

Myth	Fact
Section 135 can be used if a patient is in mental health crisis in a public place, not a private dwelling.	A police officer would use the Section 136 power if the patient is in a mental health crisis in a public place.
Section 135 can only be applied for if the patient does not have capacity.	Whether a patient has capacity or not, a warrant can be applied for. A warrant is sometimes applied for because there are concerns for the patient and no formal assessment is possible because the patient has refused to open the door.
Section 135 can only be applied for by a police officer.	Only an AMHP can apply for the warrant.
Section 135 can be used to remove a patient immediately to hospital for a medical emergency.	The Section 135 warrant specifically relates to a patient's mental health. If the patient has a medical emergency which is life-threatening, e.g. red flag sepsis, catastrophic haemorrhage etc., then reference to the Mental Capacity Act would be more appropriate.
Section 135 can only be applied for at the magistrates' court between 09.00–17.00, Monday–Friday.	A magistrate is available in every local area 24 hours a day to hear warrant applications. This may be in court or at the magistrate's home for out-of-hours applications. The AMHP will be familiar with local procedures.
Section 135 does not infringe on a patient's human rights.	Irrespective of need for a warrant, it will infringe upon a patient's human rights. Entry to their home may be forced and they will be removed to a place of safety for up to 36 hours whether they agree or not.
Section 135 provides for the detention of a patient for a period of 96 hours.	The patient will be detained for up to 36 hours. At the end of this time they could be released or detained further under the Mental Health Act, e.g. Section 2.

Mental Health Act: Section 136

Section 136 provides lawful authority for the police to remove an individual to a place of safety. They can make use of this power without a warrant when they have a reasonable belief that an individual:

- Appears to have a mental disorder
- Is not residing in a private dwelling (a house, flat or room; this includes a garden, garage or other out-building accessed by a single household; communal gardens are excluded from this definition)
- Is 'in need of immediate care or control' i.e., there is a reasonable belief that the safety of the individual or others is at risk.

Following the Policing and Crime Act 2017, police officers are obliged, where possible and practicable, to consult a registered medical practitioner, a registered nurse, an AMHP, an occupational therapist or a paramedic.

As with Section 135 detentions, the individual detained under Section 136 can then be kept at the place of safety for up to 24 hours. This can be extended for a further 12 hours, but only if the individual cannot, for clinical reasons, be assessed within the initial 24 hours. The period of detention must not be extended for operational issues, for example, a lack of available beds or staff. The period of detention commences upon arrival at the place of safety, or alternatively, upon arrival of the police if onward transfer does not occur.

Prior to the Policing and Crime Act 2017, it was common for police cells to be used as a place of safety under Section 136. While it is likely in the near future to be made unlawful for adults to be detained in police cells under Section 136, as it is for children, the latest data released by the UK government (2021a) demonstrates that in 2019/20 a police station was used as a place of safety in 159 instances which is a 98% reduction since 2012/13. Currently, the police station should only ever be used as a place of safety if the individual's behaviour creates a significant risk and it is agreed by all parties engaged in the decision-making process that this is the most appropriate place. The individual should be monitored continuously and moved to an appropriate clinical setting as soon as possible. Myths surrounding this warrant are explored in Table 1.3.

Table 1.3   Myths and facts about the Section 136 warrant.

Myth	Fact
May be used if a patient is in mental health crisis in a private dwelling.	A police officer would use the Section 135 power if the patient is in a mental health crisis in a private dwelling; this includes gardens, garages and outbuildings attached to that property.
Individuals can be asked to step outside of their private dwelling then can subsequently be detained.	This is coercion; individuals should not be coerced into entering a public space for the purposes of detention.

Section 2 of the Mental Health Act

Section 2 of the Mental Health Act provides lawful authority for the compulsory admission of an individual for assessment, or for assessment followed by medical treatment, for a period of up to 28 days.

The AMHP is responsible for making the application to detain and is supported in this by two medical recommendations. The AMHP must consider both the legal position and any lesser restrictive options available. One of the medical recommendations must be from a clinician who is approved under Section 12 of the Mental Health Act. This stipulates that they must have experience in the diagnosis or treatment of mental disorder. This will usually be a consultant or senior registrar psychiatrist, but a number of GPs will also hold such authority.

The clinical opinion or medical recommendations must agree that the period of detention is required in order to keep the individual or others safe and that the individual is suffering from a mental disorder the nature or degree of which warrants detention for assessment, or assessment followed by treatment. The individual has a right to appeal to the Mental Health Review Tribunal within 14 days of admission.

Section 3 of the Mental Health Act

Section 3 provides for a period of detention for treatment lasting up to six months, although this can be extended.

The individual must be considered to be suffering from a mental disorder, that is, 'any disorder or disability of the mind' (Mental Health Act 1983). Clinically recognised mental disorders include schizophrenia, bipolar disorder, anxiety or depression, as well as personality disorders, eating disorders and autistic spectrum disorders.

There are two points of clarification within the Mental Health Act:

- Learning disability – An individual with a learning disability may only be detained if they display abnormally aggressive or seriously irresponsible conduct.

- Dependence on alcohol or drugs – The Mental Health Act makes reference to dependence and does not exclude the effects of substances, such as intoxication, psychosis and delirium.

As with Section 2 the detention must be necessary to keep the individual or others safe and the treatment cannot be provided unless they are detained under this Section.

The individual may be detained for a period of six months, including the day of admission. Extension of detention can be obtained for a period of up to six months and then for a period of one year. The Responsible Clinician will need the written agreement of a second clinician in order to renew the Section 3. The second professional must be involved with the care of the individual and be able to reach independent decisions. The clinician must be experienced and have sufficient capability to make clinical decisions regarding whether the criteria by which detention is authorised continue to be met. The detained individual has the right to appeal to the Mental Health Review Tribunal within the first six months and then subsequently once a year should detention continue.

Subsequent to detention under Section 3, health and social care have a responsibility to ensure that appropriate aftercare is provided to maintain recovery and prevent further periods of detention. This requirement is detailed under Section 117.

Section 4 of the Mental Health Act

Section 4 allows for the emergency detention of an individual for the purpose of assessment for a period of up to 72 hours.

As with Section 2, the application can be made by the nearest relative or an AMHP and must be supported by one doctor. The doctor must have examined the patient within the previous 24 hours.

The recommendation for detention under Section 4 should reflect the clear urgent need and as such should not be made simply because there are difficulties associated with obtaining the second clinician required for detention under Section 2.

Where detention under Section 4 is made, a second subsequent medical recommendation from a doctor approved under Section 12 should be made within 72 hours of the initial detention. This will then allow a period of detention under Section 2. Section 4 cannot be renewed and must, as described above, be converted into a Section 2 detention.

Table 1.4 gives a comparative guide to the relevant sections of the Mental Health Act.

Table 1.4   Comparative guide.

Section 135	
Authority	Provides the lawful authority to detain a person within their own home, where they are suspected to be suffering from a mental health disorder.
Timescale	Individual may be held in a place of safety for 24 hours. In certain circumstances, this may be extended by a further 12 hours.
Purpose	Assessment.
Section 136	
Authority	Provides lawful authority for the police to detain an individual who appears to have a mental disorder and who is not in a private dwelling.
Timescale	Individual may be held in a place of safety for 24 hours. In certain circumstances, this may be extended by a further 12 hours.
Purpose	Assessment.
Section 2	
Authority	Compulsory admission of an individual for assessment for a period of up to 28 days.
Required	An AMHP and two doctors.
Section 3	
Authority	Compulsory admission of an individual for treatment for a period of up to six months, which can be extended.
Required	An AMHP and two doctors.
Section 4	
Authority	Emergency detention of an individual for assessment for a period of up to 72 hours.
Required	An AMHP and one doctor.

Mental Capacity Act (2005)

More detail will be provided within Chapter Two, however at this point it is worth noting the primary role of the Mental Capacity Act and to differentiate it from the Mental Health Act. The Mental Capacity Act 2005 sets out to provide the legal framework through which we might protect those vulnerable individuals who are not able to make their own decisions. It is decision specific, setting out the process by which individuals can be supported to make decisions about issues that impact on them. It outlines how decisions may be made, by whom and at what time. The Mental Capacity Act and the Mental Health Act should not be confused nor should it be assumed that any individual who is subject to one is automatically subject to the other. The Mental Health Act sets out to support the assessment and management of those who are deemed to be suffering or potentially suffering from a mental health disorder. The Mental Capacity Act seeks to support individuals in making individual decisions relating to their wellbeing and sets out five key principles that must be followed:

1. We must make an initial assumption that an individual has capacity until such time as a determination has been made that this is not the case. We can never assume that an individual lacks the ability to make a decision, irrespective of any disability or any temporary physical or mental state.

2. People must be supported to make decisions. Information relevant to the decision at hand must be made available or be presented in a manner which the individual can understand. This may require alternative communication methods or the delivery of information through intermediaries who are best placed to support the individual.

3. Individuals may make unwise decisions. We cannot make judgement on individual's decisions, we must simply ensure that they are able to make a decision based on the information available.

4. Any and all decisions must be made in their best interests. Sometimes complex, this process should include where possible information relevant to the individuals past preferences or declared desires.

5. Must ensure that decisions are least restrictive in nature. We must ensure that any decisions taken on behalf of an individual do not impose overly restrictive interventions. For example, an individual should not be admitted into a residential care facility if their needs can be met within the home environment.

References

Adebowale V. (2013). Independent Commission on Mental Health and Policing Report. Available at: https://www.basw.co.uk/system/files/resources/basw_22916-3_0.pdf

BASW (2014). The Role of the Social Worker in Adult Mental Health Services. Available at: https://www.basw.co.uk/resources/role-social-worker-adult-mental-health-services

Care Act 2014 (c.23). Available at: https://www.legislation.gov.uk/ukpga/2014/23/contents/enacted

Centre for Mental Health (2016). Mental health and criminal justice: Views from consultations across England and Wales. Available at: https://www.centreformentalhealth.org.uk/sites/default/files/2018-09/Centre_for_Mental_Health_MH_and_criminal_justice_PDF.pdf

College of Policing (2016). Authorised Professional Practice: Mental health. Available at: https://www.app.college.police.uk/app-content/mental-health/

England L. (2017). RCGP position statement on mental health in primary care. Primary Care Mental Health Steering Group. Royal College of General Practitioners. Available at: http://www.infocoponline.es/pdf/RCGP-PS-mental-health.pdf

HM Government and Mind (2014). About the Crisis Care Concordat. *Crisis Care Concordat Mental Health*. Available at: https://www.crisiscareconcordat.org.uk/about/

HMICFRS (2018). Policing and mental health: Picking up the pieces. Available at: https://www.justiceinspectorates.gov.uk/hmicfrs/publications/policing-and-mental-health-picking-up-the-pieces/

Human Rights Act 1998 (c.42). Available at: https://www.legislation.gov.uk/ukpga/1998/42/contents

Jarvis S. (2019). Refer Yourself to NHS Drug and Alcohol Support Services. *Patient*. Available at: https://patient.info/treatment-medication/self-referral/refer-yourself-to-nhs-drug-and-alcohol-support-services

Mental Capacity Act 2005 (c. 9). Available at: https://www.legislation.gov.uk/ukpga/2005/9/contents

Mental Health Act 1983 (c. 20). Available at: https://www.legislation.gov.uk/ukpga/1983/20/contents

Mental Health Act 2007 (c.12). Available at: https://www.legislation.gov.uk/ukpga/2007/12/contents

Mental Health Taskforce (2016). The NHS Five Year Forward View for Mental Health. Available at: https://www.england.nhs.uk/wp-content/uploads/2016/02/Mental-Health-Taskforce-FYFV-final.pdf

Metropolitan Police (2019). Force Management Statement. Available at: https://www.met.police.uk/SysSiteAssets/media/downloads/force-content/met/about-us/bg-to-business-plan-fms-may-2019.pdf

Mind (2018). Crisis services and planning for a crisis. Available at: https://www.Mind.org.uk/information-support/guides-to-support-and-services/crisis-services/crisis-teams-crhts/

Mind (2019). Understanding CAMHS for young people. Available at: https://www.mind.org.uk/information-support/for-children-and-young-people/understanding-camhs/

NHS (2021). Integrating mental health therapy into primary care. Available at: https://www.england.nhs.uk/mental-health/adults/iapt/integrating-mental-health-therapy-into-primary-care/

NICE (2018). Chapter 23. Liaison psychiatry, emergency and acute medical care in over 16s: service delivery and organisation. Guideline 94. Available at: https://www.nice.org.uk/guidance/ng94/evidence/23.liaison-psychiatry-pdf-172397464636

Pettit B. et al. (2013). Summary: At risk, yet dismissed: the criminal victimisation of people with mental health problems. Available at: https://www.mind.org.uk/media-a/4308/at-risk-yet-dismissed-summary.pdf

Policing and Crime Act 2017 (c.3). Available at: https://www.legislation.gov.uk/ukpga/2017/3/contents/enacted

Rethink Mental Illness (2021a). Advice and information on living with mental illness. Available at: https://www.rethink.org/advice-and-information/living-with-mental-illness/treatment-and-support/

Rethink Mental Illness (2021b). Getting help in a crisis. Available at: https://www.rethink.org/advice-and-information/carers-hub/getting-help-in-a-crisis/

Rethink Mental Illness (2021c). Criminal Justice. Available at: https://www.rethink.org/help-in-your-area/services/criminal-justice/

Royal College of Psychiatrists: Baugh C., Blanchard E. and Hopkins I. (2020) Psychiatric Liaison Accreditation Network (PLAN), Quality Standards for Liaison Psychiatry Services, Sixth Edition. Available at: https://www.rcpsych.ac.uk/docs/default-source/improving-care/ccqi/quality-networks/psychiatric-liaison-services-plan/quality-standards-for-liaison-psychiatry-services---sixth-edition-20209b6be47cb0f249f697850e1222d6b6e1.pdf?sfvrsn=1ddd53f2_0

Together for Mental Wellbeing (2021). Criminal Justice Services. Available at: https://www.together-uk.org/our-mental-health-services/criminal-justice-mental-health/

UK Government (2021a). Statutory guidance: Care and support statutory guidance. Available at: https://www.gov.uk/government/publications/care-act-statutory-guidance/care-and-support-statutory-guidance

Chapter 2

Decision Making

David Partlow

> ### Case study
>
> You have been dispatched to a healthcare professional admission call for a patient who has been assessed as lacking capacity and who requires conveyance to an emergency department.
>
> On arrival, you receive a handover from the nurse in the rapid response team who informs you that the patient is an 82-year-old male who has not engaged with his own GP. He is living alone in dirty conditions and will not allow carers to enter the property to assist him.
>
> **Assessment:**
>
> - Past medical history: hypertension, high cholesterol, coronary artery disease, right bundle branch block and transient ischaemic attack (six years previously).
> - Allergies: penicillin.
> - Drug history: ramipril, aspirin, simvastatin.
> - Social history: lives in own home, patient's wife of 50 years died five years ago, no regular family visits, carer once daily, independent in his daily activities.
>
> **On examination:**
>
> - Appearance: unkempt, wearing visibly dirty clothing contaminated with faeces. There is an overpowering and unpleasant smell within the patient's home.
> - Behaviour: patient witnessed drinking milk from the bottle that is obviously beyond the use-by date. Despite trying to reason with the patient, he continues to drink it. Carer's notes indicate concerns about changes in the patient's behaviour.
> - Speech: normal speech.

- Mood/thoughts: appears annoyed, the patient says he does not understand what all the fuss is about and is asking everyone to leave. He has stated he will not answer the door again to anyone because of this situation.
- Affect: not able to assess as patient does not cooperate.
- Perception: not able to assess as patient does not cooperate.
- Cognition: not able to assess as patient does not cooperate.
- Insight: not able to assess as patient does not cooperate.
- Risk: low risk to immediate harm.

Clinical observations:

- Heart rate: 62 beats/min; regular and equal bilaterally
- Blood pressure: 142/84 mmHg
- Blood glucose: 6.5 mml/l
- Respiratory rate: 19 breaths/min
- Temperature: 36.9°C
- SpO_2: 98% on room air

The patient agrees to you undertaking a set of observations. All observations are within normal ranges and there are no physical health clinical concerns from your findings. The information from the scene indicates evidence of self-neglect. The patient has no medical complaints. The patient does not consent to being assessed at the emergency department.

The Health Care Professional (HCP) says that the patient does not have capacity. They have a document indicating this and you are asked to convey the patient to the emergency department. You ask the HCP which section of the Mental Capacity Act he is using to legally convey the patient who does not consent to transport and admission to an emergency department and he replies, 'the patient does not have capacity, they are required to be conveyed under the Mental Capacity Act'.

What would you do now?

1. **Convey the patient against their will:** this would be unlawful as the patient would be deprived of their liberty. The Supreme Court of the United Kingdom (2014) makes clear that within the Mental Capacity Act a patient can only be deprived of their liberty (Section 4B) 'in order to give life-sustaining treatment or to prevent a serious deterioration in the person's condition while a case is pending before the court [of protection]' (see *P v Cheshire West and Chester Council and another*, 2014). You have clinically assessed the patient and find that there are no life-threatening features, for example, severe sepsis.

Point to note: if the patient does not have capacity and if there is no evidence of the need for life sustaining treatment, then a paramedic has no legal power to convey the patient against their will.

2. **Respect the patient's wishes and leave:** you have a duty of care for the patient and there are concerns about the patient's welfare including evidence of self-neglect. You must respect the patient's wishes but you have a duty to safeguard the patient. You should consult the patient's GP or make a referral to social services for the patient's welfare subject to the patient's informed consent (Care Act, 2014). The patient has declined any referrals.

   As it has been determined through an assessment of the individual's ability to understand information relevant to the decision and to retain that information, use this knowledge to make a decision and communicate it: that they do not have capacity and therefore you can act in the patient's best interests (Principle 4, Mental Capacity Act) and consult their GP. Follow your local policies and procedures for safeguarding.

3. **Refer to an Approved Mental Health Professional (AMHP):** information gleaned from the patient's home and the HCP indicates that the patient may require a mental health assessment. There are AMHPs 24 hours daily. Speak to the AMHP clinician to clinician and discuss your concerns and findings. If the AMHP agrees, they could apply for the warrant or use the Mental Health Act as appropriate.

   Section 135 of the Mental Health Act 1983 states:

   > 'If it appears to a Justice of the Peace [magistrate], on information on oath laid by an approved mental health professional, that there is reasonable cause to suspect that a person believed to be suffering from mental disorder –
   >
   > a. has been, or is being, ill-treated, neglected or kept otherwise than under proper control, in any place within the jurisdiction of the justice, or
   >
   > b. being unable to care for [them]self, is living alone in any such place' the Justice of the Peace may issue a warrant authorising any police officer to enter, if need be by force, any premises specified in the warrant in which that person is believed to be, and, if thought fit, to remove [them] to a place of safety with a view to the making of an application in respect of [them] under Part II of this Act [mental health assessment], or of other arrangements for [their] treatment or care.'

   Remember only an AMHP can apply for the Section 135 warrant.

   Justin Honey-Jones

The complexity of decision making

The scenario described above may be familiar to many who read it, and there are many others that are equally challenging and prompt many a conversation in the crew room. They outline exactly why many paramedics struggle with the decision-making process with respect to attendance at mental health presentations.

As in the scenario above, we all have a right to live the life we choose; this doesn't mean that each life has to be lived in the same way or with the same core principles. We choose how we live and we choose in some cases how we die. Professionals must use their judgement coupled with knowledge of legal frameworks to make the best decision possible for the patient.

Decision making and values-based practice is therefore about balance; it is about looking at the need for action and intervention and balancing that against the wishes of the individual and the legal context within which those decisions might need to be based.

It is necessary to employ the least restrictive interventions without utilising the legal frameworks to achieve an aim that is not supported by codes of practice or case law that has developed over time. For example, the historic practice of encouraging individuals to step out of their homes in order for them to be detained within a public space is now deemed coercive and unjustifiable under the law.

In the case of *Sessay v South London and Maudsley NHS Foundation Trust* (2011), an individual was detained and conveyed to an emergency department under the Mental Capacity Act, despite there being no threat to life or serious threat to their physical state. They were subsequently assessed under the Mental Health Act and lawfully detained. The issue, however, arose as to whether the initial conveyance under the Mental Capacity Act was lawful or a breach of the individual's rights under Article 5 of the Human Rights Act. Fundamental to this case was the provision to detain under Section 4 of the Mental Health Act and the absence of any clinical factors that warranted conveyance to an emergency department. It was deemed unacceptable to convey the individual under the auspices of the Mental Capacity Act without an emergency need. This was particularly relevant because the power to assess and detain as appropriate was already within the provision of the Mental Health Act.

Decision making is complex. Individuals responding alone without knowledge of the legal complexities or a wider understanding of mental health presentations, face a very difficult task in making a determination of the most appropriate course of action. However, mental health is no different to physical health. The decision to transfer to a place where assessment and care can be provided should be made on the basis of what assessments or interventions may be required, who is best able to deliver them and whether they are required now or at a later point in time.

Fundamental then, is the generation of an understanding in the local area of what services are available to support those in crisis. Many areas are now generating single points of contact or single points of access. A myriad of crisis cafes and respite provision are being created and as paramedics it is vital that we understand how to access such services where available and determine eligibility criteria.

First and foremost, consider the ability of an individual to consent to assessment or intervention. Consider the requirements of the Mental Capacity Act and whether there is a physical imperative that supports immediate conveyance. Work with other professionals, understand the mental health service provision and, importantly, get to know your local AMHP service. AMHPs should be consulted for their specific professional expertise on aspects of assessment and the complexities of law.

As clinicians who frequently work in an autonomous manner, it is always advisable to seek the advice of others who may have specialist knowledge that may assist in the assessment and management of any individual.

Assess the risk, engage others if possible in the decision-making process, document the decision-making process very clearly, not just the decision, consider what you plan to do and record what has been excluded and why. Never base clinical decisions on assumptions and think carefully through the likely and possible implications of the decisions you make.

Restraint

The Mental Capacity Act 2005 defines restraint as occurring when an individual 'uses, or threatens to use force to secure the doing of an act which the person resists, or restricts a person's liberty whether or not they are resisting'. This may take the form of mechanical restraint whereby a physical device is used to restrict the movement of an individual. This could take the form of straps, belts or any other device which impedes the free movement of an individual. This may be through the application of physical force, holding an individual down or by sitting on or applying physical force to restrict free movement. This may be through the application or administration of a pharmacological substance to immobilise, sedate or otherwise impede the ability of an individual to move. However, it might also be through the use of coercive language (or threat); while this form of psychological restraint might be more subtle in form, it is as restrictive as physical force and would, therefore, constitute a form of restraint.

Language is important here as organisations seeking to avoid difficult and complex subjects may prefer to use terms such as 'safe holding' to minimise the significance of any physical intervention. It is important that we understand and appreciate that any form of restrictive intervention that impedes the free movement of an individual is, in fact, restraint and as such must be managed in accordance with the appropriate legislation and the fundamental principles that should be applied to any restrictive intervention or episode of restraint. Alternative terminology does not remove the need to ensure that restrictive interventions are managed appropriately, nor does it remove organisational responsibility to ensure that staff are appropriately trained and educated.

As an absolute principle, restraint should only be applied as a last resort. Inappropriate, poorly applied restrictive interventions have been seen to cause significant harm, both physically and emotionally, and as a leading cause of deaths while in police custody.

Legal position

In certain circumstances, where the immediate situation and the potentially serious consequences of inaction dictate, common law does allow for the application of restraint in order to take immediate control of a dangerous situation. For example, when there is potential for serious harm to occur if no action is undertaken, if perhaps an individual is threatening to jump from a bridge. In such circumstances, it is acceptable to act on the belief that it is more likely than not that the individual lacks the capacity to make a decision and it is therefore best to take immediate action to restrain in order to preserve life. However, with all cases where restraint is applied it must be appropriate in character, proportionate to the risks involved and applied for the least possible time (NICE, 2015).

The Mental Capacity Act enables actions to be taken in a person's best interests where they lack capacity, for example, where restraint is needed to save the patient's life or prevent significant deterioration, and force used must be proportionate to the likely seriousness of harm to the patient. Again, restraint must be appropriate in character, proportionate to the risks involved and applied for the least possible time.

Restraint is permitted only if the person using it has reasonable belief that it is required to prevent harm to the incapacitated person, and if the restraint used is proportionate to the likelihood and seriousness of the harm. Section 6 (5) of the Mental Capacity Act is very clear in that the provision of restraint and any subsequent deprivation of liberty cannot be an action for which Section 5 provides any legal protection. Section 5 of the Mental Capacity Act makes it very clear that clinical interventions can be undertaken to support the care and treatment of an individual who lacks capacity, but that this must be on the basis of a detailed assessment of capacity and best interests.

The Mental Health Act (1983) further provides for the application of restraint to support those who are lawfully detained or liable to be detained against their wishes. It must be noted here though that while police officers can use restraint in order to enforce admission under Section 6 of the Mental Health Act, police officers must make the determination and cannot be compelled to do so.

The provision of restraint is therefore lawful under certain circumstances but is fraught with complications and must therefore be used with extreme caution.

Restraint should only be used:

- When absolutely necessary and when all other measures including communication, engagement and de-escalation have been exhausted

- In order to deliver clinical interventions necessary to save the patient's life or to prevent significant deterioration and be in their best interests

- Proportionately to the risk of harm

- In a form which is as minimally restrictive as possible

- With minimum force for the shortest period possible.

It is also vital that clear and detailed documentation is kept to record the episode of restraint, with a clear rationale for its application, the method used and the associated timings to demonstrate when it was applied and released.

Risk Factors

Due to the physical nature of restraint a number of risk factors are associated and should always be considered.

Foremost is the absolute requirement to avoid prone restraint, this places a physical restriction on the mechanisms of respiration and can lead to positional asphyxia (Department of Health, 2014). It is the responsibility of the clinician to not only ensure that they do not use prone restraint, but that they also intervene whenever it is used by others. It is important to note that the clinical responsibility for the health and welfare of the individual remains with the lead clinician, irrespective of whether they, or others, are responsible for the application of restrictive interventions.

In addition, should the individual subject to any restrictive intervention be under the influence of alcohol and/or any other substance, the impact of this on the individual must be carefully considered. It is never sufficient to consider the current level of intoxication or to ascertain what has been drunk at initial presentation. Alcohol is absorbed at different rates, based on size, weight, gender and a range of other factors. Levels of intoxication rise over time and therefore an individual may become far more intoxicated even after they have stopped drinking.

Children

When considering the provision of any restraint or restrictive intervention in children, as with adults, any actions taken must be appropriate, proportionate and applied in the least restrictive manner for the shortest period possible.

While the Mental Capacity Act does not apply to children under 16 years old, children can consent to clinical interventions when they have been assessed as being capable of making a reasoned decision.

The paramedic will need to take into consideration a number of factors when assessing a child's capacity to consent, including:

- The child's age and maturity.

- The child's understanding of the proposed intervention, including what it might deliver alongside key risks both short and long term.

- The ability of the child to understand the information provided and to use this to formulate and express an opinion,

- The child's ability to understand alternative options that may be available.

It is important to note that consent is not valid if any form of coercion is applied and that a parent cannot override the decision of a Gillick-competent child (NSPCC, 2020). This means that a child under the age of 16 can consent to their treatment if they are believed to possess sufficient intelligence, competence and an understanding of what's involved in their treatment. It is though very important to include parents in the decision-making process and particularly so when a child is deemed as not being competent.

De-escalation

Throughout the process of de-escalation it is vital that you consider the needs of the individual and that you are conversant with the methods you use to communicate, verbally or otherwise. If an individual is in crisis and suffering from significant issues of self-esteem and self-worth they may perhaps be angry or belligerent. Responding in a similar way merely reinforces that sense of self-loathing and negative self-image in the individual. It is therefore important when communicating with patients in crisis that reflecting negativity is avoided, that the paramedic uses a calm, reassuring tone, is non-judgemental and takes time to acknowledge the pain that the individual is experiencing.

The College of Policing (2020) describes the use of Betari's Box: the mechanism by which we are affected by the way we respond to others. It proposes that if we adjust our behaviour, it will in turn support adjustments in others' behaviour towards us (Figure 2.1). The core principle behind Betari's box is that we have free will in terms of how we interact with others, and therefore, we can choose to be positive, irrespective of how others are behaving towards us or how we might be feeling inwardly.

In this way, our attitude affects our behaviour which in turn affects our attitude and so the cycle continues. In simple terms, when we feel negative, we behave in a negative way towards others. Negative thoughts trigger negative behaviour, whether consciously or otherwise. This may take the form of verbalised behaviours but can also be demonstrated in non-verbal ways through body language or demeanour. Conversely, positive thoughts trigger positive behaviour. Again, this may be demonstrated in a verbal or non-verbal way.

Our behaviours, whether negative or positive, are then reflected in those we interact with and subsequently, their reaction is reflected back to us. We can therefore become

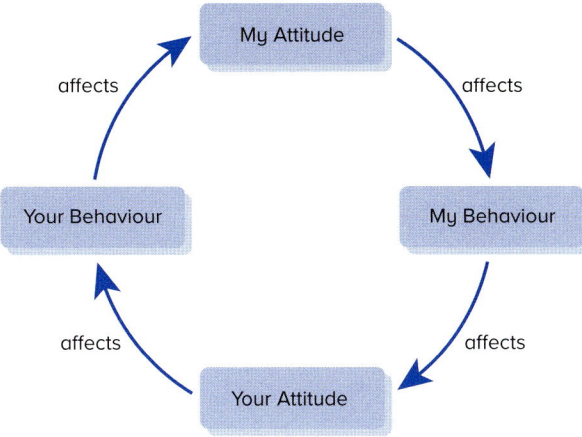

Figure 2.1 Betari's box.

stuck in a cyclical pattern of behaviour and if we can consciously change our attitude, we can break the cycle and regain control.

Understanding how our attitude can impact on the behaviour of others is therefore crucial; we must first be aware of how we are feeling and ensure that our behaviour is controlled and does not become a mere reflection of our thoughts. When confronted by negativity, we can choose to respond in kind or to take control of our attitude and behaviours to break the negative cycle and stop it from developing.

Relating this back to the initial Case Study, we must consider how our approach may need to be adapted to ensure that we do not create a negative cycle in our engagement with the individual who has not previously accepted support from his GP or agreed to attempts by healthcare professionals to enter his premises to support him. Communication is key, as is the degree of empathy with which we approach the situation. Understanding the needs, and fears of this individual is an important first step in supporting them to make an informed decision and allaying the fears and concerns that they may have which may be creating a barrier to accepting the help that is being offered.

Suicide

Unfortunately, as paramedics we will be called upon to attend incidents that involve attempts by individuals to end their own life. We will also be called to verify or recognise death in such circumstances. In 2019, 5,691 people took their own life in England and Wales (ONS, 2019). Approximately three-quarters of registered deaths were men (4,303 deaths) with a male suicide rate of 16.9 deaths per 100,000 which is the highest rate since 2000.

While this book is focused on mental health, it is important to note that over 65% of those who die by suicide are not known to mental health services. While an important factor, suicide of itself is not a mental health issue and activities associated with prevention must be based on a broader consideration of factors associated with socioeconomic deprivation.

Risk factors

There are a number of risk factors associated with suicide which should be considered during any assessment (Harding, 2019). These include where an individual (Harris, 2018):

- Has made previous attempts to end their life

- Has a family history of suicide

- Has been diagnosed with mental health problems

- Has recently been discharged from psychiatric hospital (the first week and in particular, the first three days are a particularly high risk period)

- Is socially isolated, this is particularly important when considering social isolation in the elderly

- Has been unemployed for more than one month, this is particularly important when periods of economic hardship occur through recession or in response for example, to the COVID-19 pandemic

- Is homeless (The Office for National Statistics data for 2017 showed that 13% of deaths among homeless people were due to suicide and that suicide was the second most common cause of death for homeless people)

- Has a debilitating or terminal illness.

- Identifies as LGBTQ2+. While national data is not held it is widely accepted that members of the LGBTQ2+ community experience a significantly higher risk of suicide.

There is also a strong correlation and link between physical and mental health. Just as poor physical health can lead to a deterioration in mental health, the opposite is equally true.

Those suffering from mental ill-health are far less likely to receive treatment or to be in receipt of any formal physical health assessment; they are also less likely to self-present to health services and are therefore much less likely to have underlying conditions identified at an early stage. Consequently, they are less likely to receive help with poor lifestyle choices and more likely to smoke, consume alcohol and have a less healthy diet.

There are also significant correlations around social inequity and deprivation, both in terms of increasing the associated risk factors for both poor physical and mental health and also in respect of fewer opportunities to access services that may assist in providing effective intervention.

It is, therefore, far too complex to suggest that poor physical health creates the environment in which poor mental health can flourish, or whether it is the other way around, but we can say that one cannot be considered without the other.

While some suicides may appear to be spontaneous, and leave loved ones with significant feelings of anguish and despair, others follow a change in behaviour in the individual over a period of time (Rethink Mental Health, 2021).

- Expressions of hopelessness or helplessness – it is incredibly difficult for individuals who are struggling with their mental health to be able to see any positives in life or any hope for the future.

- An overwhelming sense of shame or guilt – many individuals feel that they have low worth and with that, a real sense of being weak and less able than others.

- A dramatic change in personality or appearance – many individuals begin to outwardly reflect how they feel about themselves and their worth. Giving up washing, shaving, or concern for outward appearance – in essence, mirroring in appearance how they perceive themselves to be.

- Behaving 'out of character' – behaving in a way that they would not ordinarily do.

- Altered eating or sleeping habits. An inability to sleep and reduction in appetite leading to weight loss is common.

- A serious decline in college or work performance – this could be due to an inability to concentrate or through a belief that work or performance no longer matter.

- A lack of interest in the future – a clear inability to see a time when things will be better may be present.

- Written or spoken notice of intention to end own life – this would clearly be a significant concern and may indicate a significant escalation in the level of risk.

- Giving away possessions or putting affairs in order – may indicate a finalisation of planning.

- Sudden unexplained 'recovery' – some individuals may appear positive when they have made the final decision to end their life, the pain and anguish are sometimes lifted as the individual is at peace with the decision. This may then be reflected with a sudden positive improvement in appearance and behaviour without any perceived reason.

It is important to stress that the risks, and associated behavioural changes, may not always be present; it is therefore vital that we encourage conversations around mental health and suicide, such that it becomes OK to *not* be OK and it becomes OK to ask for help.

Communication

For paramedics, the determination of risk is incredibly important and phrasing a conversation with an individual who may be considering, or may have attempted to take their own life, is a crucial part of that assessment.

We, as paramedics have probably all heard colleagues state that they 'don't know what to say' in these situations, when in reality they often just need to listen and to try to understand.

The following is a suggested framework for conversations; it is not a checklist and should not be used as such. When discussing suicide with an individual in distress, it is important that the conversation happens in a safe environment in a way and at a pace that meets the needs of the individual.

Suicide is complex; suggested changes in behaviour may or may not be present, therefore making a determination of the associated risk is incredibly difficult and any tool used to support the evaluation of risk must be used carefully. When assessing the level of risk it is important to consider four factors: intent, plans, actions and protective measures. These factors form the IPAP Suicide Risk Assessment Tool which can be used by a non-mental health professional to identify and assess suicidal risk (Table 2.1). The IPAP assessment tool should be used to help inform immediate management on scene, not as part of a long-term measure of the patient's condition (JRCALC, 2019). This tool forms part of a wider holistic assessment of the individual and should be used to inform the decision making along with other pertinent factors which may increase the risk of suicide.

> **Remember!**
>
> Suicidal thoughts are not always rational, but that does not in any way mean that those concerns and beliefs are not very real. Suicide is not always about ending life; it can also be about ending pain.

The important point to make here is that for a person in crisis, conversation, human kindness and empathy are important and taking time to make a difference is also important.

- It's OK to ask
- Being that person who cares is all it may take
- You are not going to make it worse by caring.

Further resources are available from the National Suicide Prevention Alliance at https://www.nspa.org.uk/ and the Zero Suicide Alliance at https://www.zerosuicidealliance.com/

Table 2.1 IPAP suicide risk assessment tool.

Intent	• When trying to evaluate the level of intent, ask the individual if they are feeling suicidal. A myth exists that asking this question somehow increases the likelihood that they will subsequently complete the act of taking their own life. This is simply not true, asking the question is vital in understanding whether the individual has had or is currently suffering from suicidal thoughts. • Ask how intrusive the thoughts are. Do the thoughts come and go? Are they pervasive? Do they think about suicide daily? Are they unable to experience periods of time when the thoughts are not present? • Ask the individual whether they have thought about suicide previously; if so, what stopped them from following through with those thoughts? If they have made previous attempts, ask about those attempts and when they occurred.
Plans	• If the individual has a clear intent, the level of risk is clearly increasing; it is then important to understand whether the individual has developed a plan by which they would take their own life. • Again, it is OK to have that conversation. Asking an individual about their plans is a vital part of the dialogue and does not in itself increase the risk. • Ask the individual if they have formulated a plan and what that plan might be. Is the plan realistic and fully formed such that it could be carried out?
Actions	• If the individual has clear intent and a formulated and viable plan, the level of risk is again increased. • It is then important to understand what actions, if any, have been taken towards completion of the plan. Has the individual written any letters or closed bank accounts? Have they taken action to put their affairs in order? • Has the individual taken actions to advance the plan? Have they stockpiled medications? Have they purchased items that would be required to carry out the plan or otherwise taken actions to ensure that the plan can be activated?
Protective measures (LACK of these increases risk)	• Finally, consider protective measures and preventative factors. If the individual has considered suicide in the past, what stopped them? Is that factor still in existence or has there been a change in the individual's support network? • Does the individual have coping mechanisms or a support network? Don't be judgemental about what this may consist of. For some, the protective measure may be family or friends, but for others this will not be the case. For many, family is a significant part of the disordered thoughts of the individual, in that they truly believe loved ones will be better off without them. They may also feel that they are the source of personal or financial problems and therefore believe that by ending their life they are removing the source of the problem.

Note: always consider the above in conjunction with other known risk factors such as age, gender, employment status and significant life events (e.g. relationship breakdown, divorce, bereavement, childbirth, unemployment or economic difficulties).

Source: informed by the *JRCALC Clinical Guidelines*, 2019.

Suicide bereavement

Bereavement of any kind is painful; loss is difficult to come to terms with and emotions and grief are difficult to deal with. Loss through suicide is acknowledged as being particularly complex. Emotions associated with the loss are combined with a sense of shock and an inability to comprehend why it has happened. For some, this comes with feelings of guilt or shame and an inability to talk or communicate with those who have a shared understanding of loss through suicide (McDonnell et al., 2020).

Stigma associated with loss by suicide may lead to individuals feeling isolated; they may also wish to deny that they have been bereaved through suicide through shame or cultural religious beliefs (Pitman et al., 2018).

It is, therefore, an important role of paramedics who attend at the point of death to manage the initial interaction with loved ones, to support them as they struggle to come to terms with what has happened and to ensure that they consider the needs of those left behind. Paramedics must be mindful that they are present at the best and at the worst of times. As such, what they say and do is incredibly impactful and will stay with the bereaved for the rest of their lives.

Supportive organisations and useful contacts

- Suicide Bereavement UK: https://suicidebereavementuk.com/
- Survivors of Bereavement by Suicide: https://uksobs.org/
- Losing someone to Suicide (MIND): https://www.mind.org.uk/information-support/guides-to-support-and-services/bereavement/bereavement-by-suicide/
- Cruse Bereavement Support: https://www.cruse.org.uk/understanding-grief/grief-experiences/traumatic-loss/coping-when-someone-dies-by-suicide/
- Samaritans: https://www.samaritans.org/about-samaritans/research-policy/bereavement-suicide-services/
- Support After Suicide Partnership: https://supportaftersuicide.org.uk/

References

College of Policing (2013). Authorised Professional Practice. Detention and custody: Control, restraint and searches. Available at: https://www.app.college.police.uk/app-content/detention-and-custody-2/control-restraint-and-searches/

College of Policing (2020). Conflict management skills. Available at: https://www.college.police.uk/guidance/conflict-management/conflict-management-skills

Department of Health (2014). Positive and Proactive Care: reducing the need for restrictive interventions. Available at: https://assets.publishing.service.gov.uk/government/uploads/system/uploads/attachment_data/file/300293/JRA_DoH_Guidance_on_RP_web_accessible.pdf

Harding M. (2019). Suicide Risk Assessment and Threats of Suicide. *Patient.* Available at: https://patient.info/doctor/suicide-risk-assessment-and-threats-of-suicide

Harris J. (2018). Beyond the Horizon – A Reflection on LGBT Suicide. *LGBT foundation*. Available at: https://lgbt.foundation/news/beyond-the-horizon---a-reflection-on-lgbt-suicide/220

Joint Royal Colleges Ambulance Liaison Committee; Association of Ambulance Chief Executives (2019) *JRCALC Clinical Guidelines 2019*. Bridgwater: Class Professional Publishing.

McDonnell S. et al. (2020). Support After Suicide Partnership Report 2020. From Grief to Hope: The Collective Voice of Those Bereaved by Suicide in the UK. Available at: https://suicidebereavementuk.com/wp-content/uploads/2020/11/From-Grief-to-Hope-Report.pdf

Mind (2013). Mental health crisis care: physical restraint in crisis. A report on physical restraint in hospital settings. Available at: https://www.Mind.org.uk/media-a/4378/physical_restraint_final_web_version.pdf

Mind (2019). Bereavement. Available at: https://www.Mind.org.uk/information-support/guides-to-support-and-services/bereavement/bereavement-by-suicide/

National Survivor User Network (NSUN) and Mind (2015). Restraint in mental health services: What the guidance says. Available at: https://www.Mind.org.uk/media-a/4429/restraintguidanceweb1.pdf

NICE (2015). Violence and aggression: short-term management in mental health, health and community settings, NICE guideline [NG10]. Available at: https://www.nice.org.uk/guidance/ng10/chapter/1-recommendations

NSPCC Learning (2020). Gillick competency and Fraser guidelines. Available at: https://learning.nspcc.org.uk/child-protection-system/gillick-competence-fraser-guidelines

Office for National Statistics (2019). Suicides in England and Wales: 2019 registrations. Available at: https://www.ons.gov.uk/peoplepopulationandcommunity/birthsdeathsandmarriages/deaths/bulletins/suicidesintheunitedkingdom/2019registrations

P (by his litigation friend the Official Solicitor) (Appellant) v Cheshire West and Chester Council and another (Respondents) [2014] EWCA Civ 1257, 2011 EWCA Civ 190. Available at: https://www.supremecourt.uk/cases/docs/uksc-2012-0068-judgment.pdf

Pitman A.L., Stevenson F., Osborn D.P.J. and King M.B. (2018). The stigma associated with bereavement by suicide and other sudden deaths: A qualitative interview study. *Social Science and Medicine*, 198: 121–129.

R (Sessay) v South London and Maudsley NHS Foundation Trust [2011] EWHC 2617 (QB). Available at: https://www.mentalhealthlaw.co.uk/R_(Sessay)_v_South_London_and_Maudsley_NHS_Foundation_Trust_(2011)_EWHC_2617_(QB)

Rethink Mental Health (2021). Suicidal thoughts – How to support someone. Available at: https://www.rethink.org/advice-and-information/carers-hub/suicidal-thoughts-how-to-support-someone/

Part 2

Management of Mental Health Conditions

Chapter 3

Depression

Ursula Rolfe

Case study

You are working as a paramedic prescriber in primary care. Your second patient of the day is a 42-year-old man. He is attending alone, and you note from his records that he is rarely seen in general practice, having had a consultation a year ago for a sprained ankle. His records indicate he is a non-smoker who drinks around 20 units during the week. He had a private 'well man' check through his employer six months ago but did not mention his low mood.

He tells you he is attending because he feels he is depressed and that it is getting worse. He broke up with his girlfriend around two years ago and feels this started around then, although he feels he has moved on from that relationship. He has tried a few 'self-help' books and mobile phone apps but doesn't feel these have helped him at all. When undertaking a self-test using the Patient Health Questionnaire – 9 (PHQ-9) app on his phone, he says he keeps scoring between 17 and 22 and the app advised he talk to a healthcare professional. He has stopped playing for his local football and darts teams as he was no longer enjoying these sessions and felt like he was a bit of a failure at all sports. His sleep has been worse the last few months, with frequent early morning waking around 04.00 hours, and he is unable to go back to sleep.

Assessment

- Past medical history: rarely consults in primary care; sprained ankle one year ago.
- Allergies: no known drug allergies.
- Drug history: occasional multivitamins.
- Social history: lives alone. Works as a data analyst for a large logistics company.
- Forensic history: nil.
- Laboratory results: from a private medical 'well man' check show normal bloods including FBC, U+Es, HbA1C, LFTs and TFTs.

On examination

- Appearance: he appears unshaven this morning. He is wearing clothes which appear to be un-ironed but clean. His dress is appropriate for a visit to the GP.
- Behaviour: his behaviour is generally appropriate during the consultation, with fairly good eye contact. His posture appears introverted with moderate psychomotor retardation.
- Speech: his speech is of a low volume and fairly monotone. He is appropriately responsive to questions.
- Mood: he feels his mood is low and on further questioning describes features of anhedonia.
- Affect: he appears blunted in affect.
- Thought: on questioning, no formal thought disorders are identified. Form, content and possession appear normal.
- Perception: no disorders of perception are identified.
- Cognition: you do not formally assess his cognition; however, it appears intact during your conversation.
- Insight and judgement: he has clear insight that something is wrong and is eager to seek help and try treatments. He feels he is not himself and that he has a depressive illness.
- Risk: he describes fleeting thoughts of suicide, specifically hanging, but has no firm plans nor has he undertaken any preparatory work. He denies deliberate self-harm. You note a few additional clear risk factors: he is a single, middle-aged man with moderate alcohol use.

Clinical observations

- Heart rate: 78 beats/min
- Blood pressure: 138/96 mmHg
- Blood glucose: 5.2 mml/l
- Respiratory rate: 16 breaths/min
- Temperature: 36.8°C
- SpO_2: 99% on room air

Impression

Moderate depression

Questions for consideration

- What are some possible physiological/pathological causes of this man's symptoms?
- How do you assess a patient's risk of suicide? (Do you use any quantitative tools)?
- How do you discuss the initiation of SSRI medications, and what initial follow-up do you arrange?

Plan

Referral for online cognitive behavioural therapy (CBT) for depression. You briefly discuss that reducing his alcohol intake and increasing his exercise may be beneficial. You decide an antidepressant may be useful here and prescribe citalopram 20 milligrams once a day, after discussing this with the patient. You arrange a review appointment in two weeks to discuss any side effects and a further appointment in six weeks to review his low mood. You ensure the patient is aware of avenues for seeking further help both routinely and in crisis.

In this case, the patient is presenting with a range of signs and symptoms which point towards a diagnosis of a depressive illness. His anhedonia, low mood, sleep disturbance, psychomotor retardation, suicidal ideation and feelings of worthlessness would be enough to consider this a moderate depression. A multimodal approach to treatment is warranted here. In this case that includes advice around alcohol consumption and exercise, a referral for cognitive behavioural therapy and the initiation of pharmacological therapy. In cases such as this, a clear plan for follow-up and appropriate safety-netting are also essential.

Tom Mallinson

Patient voice

'Just because I am depressed doesn't mean I am vulnerable. I have good days and bad days but this doesn't make me abnormal'

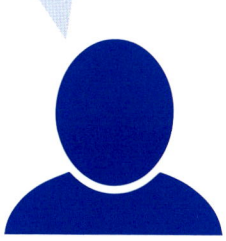

Do not do ...

- Do not recommend varying treatment strategies for depression

- Be aware of drug interactions with patients on antidepressant medications

- Medication management should not be a separate intervention and is more effective as part of a more complex intervention (NICE, 2020)

- Do not prescribe or advise patients to take St John's Wort due to uncertainty about appropriate doses, effects and potentially serious interactions with other drugs (NICE, 2020)

Recognising depression

Depression is one of the most common mental health presentations you will come across as paramedics. Recognising the condition and understanding its causes and symptoms will contribute to your management of this condition in your area of clinical expertise. According to Global Burden of Disease (2017), Chesney, Goodwin and Fazel (2014) and Correll et al. (2017), depression is one of the principal causes of disability worldwide and a major contributor to suicide and heart disease. Depression often presents in conjunction with other mental health presentations (McManus et al., 2014; Brent and Maalouf, 2015; and Cullen and Bornova, 2016). Patient numbers might also reflect the fact that major depression appears to be more common in women rather than men (Sadler et al., 2017).

Depression is more than just feeling low or fed up for a couple of days. According to the NHS (2019a), many people can feel down every now and then but when you are depressed, this changes to feeling persistently sad for weeks or months. If a patient has been diagnosed with depression, they may also have been categorised as having mild, moderate or severe depression. There are different types of depression: dysthymia, seasonal affective disorder, prenatal depression and postpartum depression (Mind, 2019). Dysthymia is defined as a patient having mild depression that lasts for about two or more years; it can sometimes also be referred to as persistent depressive disorder or chronic depression. On the other hand, seasonal affective disorder, or SAD, happens during a particular season, for example, in winter. Prenatal depression is prevalent during pregnancy and is sometimes also referred to as antenatal depression. Postpartum depression (PPD), also known as postnatal depression (PND), occurs in the months or weeks after becoming a parent. Interestingly, it is most often diagnosed in women, but can also be prevalent in men (Mind, 2019).

Understanding depression

There is no single cause of depression. It really depends on the individual patient but sometimes, a stressful event such as divorce, sickness, job or money concerns can cause depression (NHS, 2019b). Some studies suggest that patients are more likely to become depressed as they get older and that it is more common in those with difficult economic and/or social problems (NHS, 2019b). Some people become depressed for no obvious reason. Possible causes of depression are listed as follows (Mind, 2019):

- Other mental health presentations
- Childhood incidents
- Life experiences
- Physical health problems
- Genetics
- Medication
- Recreational drugs and alcohol
- Lack of sleep
- Poor diet
- Lack of exercise.

Other mental health issues may include eating problems, post-traumatic stress disorder and anxiety. Difficulty in dealing with these problems may trigger depression. Traumatic childhood experiences such as physical, sexual or emotional mistreatment, neglect, the loss of someone close to you, a traumatic event or a volatile family situation, are some additional examples (Mind, 2019). Life experiences, such as the end of a relationship, bereavement, being bullied or physically or sexually abused, loss of employment, major life changes, such as marriage, divorce, moving house or changing jobs can also contribute to depression (Mind, 2019). Certain personality traits (such as low self-esteem or being overly self-critical), giving birth, the use of alcohol and drugs are other possible causative factors (NHS, 2019b). Interestingly Parasole (2017) adds that an increase in competition, an individual's personality characteristics and extrinsic motivation can also play a role.

Diagnosis of depression can be complicated, and this is not the role of the paramedic. However, having the underpinning knowledge of how depression is diagnosed will help you manage your patient with better support and understanding around their condition. NHS (2019a) considers depression under three criteria: mild depression, mild to moderate depression and moderate to severe depression. NICE (2020) states that depression is diagnosed using the *Diagnostic and Statistical Manual of Mental Disorders (DSM-5)* criteria. An appropriately trained clinician will start by assessing two 'core' symptoms by asking: 'During the last month have you often been bothered by feeling down, depressed, or hopeless? And do you have little interest or pleasure in doing things?'. If these two core elements are present most days, most of the time and for at least two weeks, further questions need to be asked about other typical symptoms which include (NICE, 2020):

- Tiredness/energy loss
- Worthlessness/inappropriate guilt

- Recurrent thoughts of death

- Suicidal ideation or actual suicide attempts

- Reduced ability to think/concentrate or indecisiveness

- Psychomotor distress or hindrance

- Insomnia/hypersomnia

- Noteworthy appetite and/or weight loss.

Remember!

It is your role to consider differential diagnoses.

NICE (2020) suggests that if a patient is reacting to grief, this can be difficult to discern from depression. They add that dementia can also present as depression and vice versa and substances and adverse drug reactions can also produce 'depressive symptoms'. Finally, another differential diagnosis to consider is the presentation of hypothyroidism, which can also present as depression (NICE, 2020). There are no physical tests for depression, but a GP can further examine your patient and carry out blood and urine tests to rule out the possibility of hypothyroidism.

Self-help ideas for your patient

Remember that depression can often be a difficult experience for your patient and they may also be struggling to communicate and engage with others. It is therefore noteworthy that you can start your care of this patient with some supportive ideas to encourage their engagement in their condition. There are some tips you can suggest as well as some supportive tools which may help your patient reach out to others.

Importance of physical wellbeing

When patients experience depression, it can make it hard for them to find the energy to look after themselves. But looking after their physical health can make a difference. Often when patients experience depression they sleep too much or too little; find out the sleep pattern of your patient and suggest that developing a good sleep pattern can improve their mood and increase energy levels.

Consider the patient's diet. Eating regularly and ensuring their blood sugar remains stable is a good start. Many people may find the thought of exercise overwhelming when they are depressed, but exercises such as swimming, walking and yoga can help boost mood levels. Mind (2019) suggests that one way of keeping active is to join a group. This could be anything from joining a sports team to joining a community project or hobby group. Emphasise that your patient should choose an activity they enjoy as it helps fuel their motivation. Volunteering is another way to keep active and can help patients feel less alone. Encourage your patient to set realistic and achievable goals. Achieving these goals will help them to feel better and boost their self-confidence. Spending time in nature has been found to be helpful for patients with mental health problems like depression (Berman et al., 2012; Bragg, Wood and Barton, 2013). For example, research into ecotherapy, a type of formal treatment which involves doing activities outside in nature, has shown it can help with mild to moderate depression (Jordan and Hinds, 2016). This might be due to combining regular physical activity and social contact with being outside in nature.

Personal hygiene is easy to overlook when patients feel depressed. Suggest that taking a shower and getting fully dressed can make a difference to how they are feeling.

Reaching out to others

It might feel hard for your patient to start talking about how they are feeling, but many people find that sharing their experiences can help them feel better. It may be that just having someone listen to them and showing they care can help in itself. There are also a variety of free 24-hour telephone helplines that anyone can access for a confidential conversation.

Peer support is another way of sharing experiences and bringing people together who have had similar experiences. Many people find it helps them to share ideas about how to stay well, connect with others and feel less alone (Mind, 2019). There are a variety of support groups available to meet the needs of patients. The best way to access them is to search for specialist organisations via the internet. As a paramedic, you may also be aware of local support groups in your area.

Reflective practices for your patient

One way of bringing your patient into the present moment is called mindfulness. This helps them focus on where they are now, thus not fixating on the past or feeling anxious about the future – which often fuels depressive symptoms. Certain studies show that practising mindfulness can help to manage depression (Hofmann et al., 2010; Kuyken et al., 2016). Some structured mindfulness-based therapies have also been developed to treat these problems more formally. For example, NICE (2019b) recommends mindfulness-based cognitive therapy for the management of depression.

You could also consider advising your patient to start a mood diary. This can help them keep track of any changes in their mood and could help highlight that they may have more good days than they think. It is also useful to highlight which activities, places or people, if any, make them feel better or worse (Mind, 2019).

Clinical treatment and management

There are various treatments for depression. Our main resource for the treatment and management of depression is from NICE and the NHS website for clinical depression. These guidelines should be used in conjunction with your clinical judgement as well as local protocols and guidelines suggested by your clinical setting.

NHS (2019a) suggests that treatment is recommended according to what type of depression your patient may have: mild depression, mild to moderate depression and moderate to severe depression. Treatment will usually include a combination of self-help (p. 48), talking therapies and medicines.

Talking therapies include cognitive behavioural therapy (CBT) which aims to help the patient understand their thoughts and behaviours. CBT is available on the NHS for patients with depression. Normally a short course comprises six to eight sessions over 10 to 12 weeks on a one-to-one basis with a counsellor. In some cases, group CBT might also be offered (NHS, 2019a). Interpersonal therapy is another talking therapy that focuses on relationships and problems such as difficulty in communicating or coping with loss and bereavement. In psychodynamic psychotherapy, a psychoanalytic therapist will encourage patients to say whatever is going through their mind. This will help patients become aware of hidden meanings or patterns. Counselling is a form of talking therapy that helps patients think about the problems they have so that they can find new ways of dealing with them (NHS, 2019a). Counsellors support patients in finding new ways of dealing with things but they do not tell patients what to do. This type of talking therapy is ideal for patients who are generally healthy but are coping with a crisis such as anger, relationship issues, bereavement, redundancy, infertility or serious illness (NHS, 2019a).

From a clinical perspective, NICE (2020) divides management of depression into two categories: new, or initial, management and ongoing management. Although we are not expected to diagnose mental health conditions, it is important to have an understanding of the treatment so we can help point patients in the right direction for ongoing or initial care.

New, or initial, management

Patients with depression need a thorough assessment that doesn't just take a list of symptoms into account, but also considers functional deficiencies and/or ill health associated with depression. NICE (2020) recommends that you should take other factors into account, which could affect the development and severity of depression. According to NICE, these factors include:

- A past medical history of depression
- Other mental health issues or chronic physical disorders
- A past history of mood swings and the possibility of bipolar disorder
- Past treatments
- Interpersonal relationships and support
- Living circumstances (living alone or with others)
- Family history of mental health issues
- Past sexual abuse or domestic violence; job status and immigration status
- Availability of external support.

Cognitive impairment and learning difficulties also need to be considered. Other conditions that can exacerbate depression include:

- Alcohol or substance misuse
- Eating disorders
- Psychosis and schizophrenia and bipolar disorder
- Anxiety and dementia.

Depression questionnaires can also be helpful in detecting depression and its severity but NICE (2020) recommends that they should not be used in isolation. NICE (2020) recommends three questionnaires which are validated for primary healthcare use – PHQ-9 (Patient Health Questionnaire 9), HADS (Hospital Anxiety and Depression Scale), and BDI-II (Back Depression Inventory-II). Further information about these questionnaires can be found on the NICE clinical knowledge summaries website.

Remember!

Consider the risk of suicide, and don't be shy in asking direct questions about suicidal thoughts or intent.

NICE (2020) has clear questions to assess suicide risk. When assessing the risk of suicide, ask your patient whether they have contemplated suicide or death. Ask them whether they feel like their life is no longer worth living and whether they have tried to take their own life before this assessment. A family history of suicide may also be relevant. If your patient answers yes to any of these questions, NICE (2020) recommends you ask what their plans are for suicide in more detail, for example, have they thought of the way they would take their own life, do they have access to relevant materials to do so and have they prepared for it (e.g. written to their loved ones). Conversely, NICE (2020) also suggests asking your patient how they protect themself. For example, what stops them from harming themselves? Can they identify any positive reasons for staying alive? As clinicians we also need to be aware of the risk factors that increase the risk of suicide. These are:

- Previous attempts at self-harm or suicide
- Family history of suicide/self-harm or mental ill-health
- Active mental ill-health
- Being male
- Being jobless
- Living alone
- Other physical health issues
- Being single

- Drug and alcohol dependence
- Feeling hopeless and being exposed to suicidal behaviour.

NICE (2020) also adds that certain patients will be at higher risk; these groups include:

- Young or middle-aged males
- Patients within the criminal justice system
- Doctors
- Nurses
- Veterinary staff
- Farmers.

You can also use the IPAP tool to help guide your risk assessment, which can be found in Chapter 2 – Decision Making (p. 25).

Safeguarding remains a priority and if you feel your patient is at risk of self-harm or suicide, make sure you assess whether your patient has enough social support or is aware of external sources of support. Consider dynamic risk factors (as discussed above) and arrange support and safeguard your patient appropriately. Also, make use of your local safeguarding protocols and complete the relevant paperwork as supportive evidence.

Remember!

Don't forget to also consider and manage other conditions such as alcohol and substance misuse, anxiety, eating disorders, dementia and other psychotic disorders.

For patients with mild depression who do not want further help, ensure appropriate safety-netting and arrange a follow-up appointment (within two weeks) with their GP for active monitoring purposes. For patients with mild to moderate depression, NICE (2020) recommends low intensity psychosocial intervention or group-based cognitive behavioural therapy. Do not prescribe antidepressants if you are a supplementary and independent paramedic prescriber. NICE (2020) advises clinicians to consider antidepressants only for patients with a history of moderate to severe depression, those with depressive symptoms that have persisted for at least two years, patients with symptoms that have continued despite treatment and patients who present with mild depression but have complications such as other chronic health issues.

For patients with moderate to severe depression, NICE (2020) recommends antidepressants and high intensity psychosocial intervention via referral to

Improving Access to Psychological Therapies (IAPT). Also make sure your patient has follow-up appointments.

If a patient with depression presents with considerable immediate risk to themselves or others, refer them urgently to specialist mental health services such as crisis services. If they are considered to be at low risk, discuss and/or create a safety plan with them, detailing steps they should take if their situation deteriorates.

Ongoing management

NICE (2020) guidelines recommend that assessing and managing suicide risk is the first part of ongoing management of patients with depression as well as taking any safeguarding issues into consideration. If your patient has not responded well to initial treatment consider elevating their treatment. For patients with mild to moderate depression, consider low intensity psychosocial intervention. However, if this failed initially, consider an antidepressant or high intensity psychosocial intervention. If your patient is already taking antidepressants, ask them about their adherence and speak to their GP about increasing their dose or changing their antidepressants. For patients presenting with moderate to severe depression with no positive response to their initial treatment, again, elevate from initial management and double check adherence to initial medication and therapy suggestions. You could also refer your patient to specialist services for further assessment and intervention. Primarily, these patients require regular follow-up appointments to assess whether they are responding well to their treatment.

Often patients will ask you about antidepressants. These are medicines that treat the symptoms of depression and there are more than 30 types available (NHS, 2019a). Unless you are an independent prescriber and prescribing is included in your personal formulary, refer patients who want to discuss antidepressants to their own GP. However, it is useful to know that there are two main antidepressants prescribed by GPs.

The first types of antidepressants are called selective serotonin reuptake inhibitors (SSRIs). Examples of commonly used SSRI antidepressants are paroxetine, fluoxetine and citalopram. These SSRIs help increase the level of a natural chemical in the brain called serotonin. SSRIs work just as well as older antidepressants and have fewer side effects, although they can cause nausea, headaches, a dry mouth and problems having sex. But these side effects usually improve over time. Some SSRIs are not suitable for children and young people under 18 years of age. Research shows that the risk of self-harm, aggression and suicidal behaviour may increase if they are taken by under-18s (Sharma et al., 2016). Fluoxetine is the only SSRI that can be prescribed for under-18s and, even then, only when a specialist has given the go-ahead. Vortioxetine is an SSRI recommended by NICE for treating severe depression in adults (NHS, 2019a).

The other type of antidepressants are called tricyclic antidepressants (TCAs). These are a group of antidepressants used to treat moderate to severe depression and include imipramine (Imipramil) and amitriptyline. They raise the levels of serotonin and noradrenaline in the brain which help to lift mood. Side effects vary from person to person but may include a dry mouth, blurred vision, constipation, problems passing urine, sweating, feeling light-headed and excessive drowsiness. These side effects usually ease within 10 days as the body gets used to the medicine (NHS, 2019a).

According to NHS (2019a) there are newer antidepressants, such as venlafaxine (Efexor), duloxetine (Cymbalta or Yentreve) and mirtazapine (Zispin Soltab), which work in a slightly different way to SSRIs and TCAs. Venlafaxine and duloxetine are known as serotonin-noradrenaline reuptake inhibitors (SNRIs). Like TCAs, they change the levels of serotonin and noradrenaline in the brain.

NICE (2020) adds that antidepressants are not addictive in the same way that illegal or recreational drugs and cigarettes are, but patients may have some withdrawal symptoms which include: flu-like symptoms, digestive issues, anxiety, dizziness, vivid dreams and sensations in the body that feel like electric shocks. In most cases, these symptoms are quite mild and last no longer than one or two weeks, but occasionally they can be quite severe. According to the NHS (2019a) they seem to be most likely to occur with paroxetine (Seroxat) and venlafaxine (Efexor). Withdrawal symptoms occur very soon after stopping the tablets and are therefore easy to distinguish from symptoms of depression relapse, which tend to occur after a few weeks.

References

Berman M. et al. (2012). Interacting with nature improves cognition and affect for individuals with depression. *Journal of Affective Disorders*, 140(3): 300–305.

Bragg R., Wood C. and Barton J. (2013). Ecominds effects on mental wellbeing: An evaluation for Mind. Available at: https://www.mind.org.uk/media-a/4418/ecominds-effects-on-mental-wellbeing-evaluation-report.pdf

Brent D. and Maalouf F. (2015). Depressive disorders in childhood and adolescence. In Thapar, A. et al. (eds), *Rutter's Child and Adolescent Psychiatry*, 6th edn. Chichester: Wiley Blackwell.

Chesney E., Goodwin G.M. and Fazel S. (2014). Risks of all-cause and suicide mortality in mental disorders: a meta-review. *World Psychiatry*, 13(2): 153–160.

Correll C.U. et al. (2017). Prevalence, incidence and mortality from cardiovascular disease in patients with pooled and specific severe mental illness: a large-scale meta-analysis of 3,211,768 patients and 113,383,368 controls. *World Psychiatry*, 16(2): 163–180.

Cullen K.R. and Bortnova A. (2016). Mood disorders in children and adolescents. In *The Medical Basis of Psychiatry*, 4th edn. New York: Springer.

GBD (2017) Disease and Injury Incidence and Prevalence Collaborators. Global, regional, and national incidence, prevalence, and years lived with disability for 354 diseases and injuries for 195 countries and territories, 1990–2017: a systematic analysis for the Global Burden of Disease Study 2017, *The Lancet*, 392(10159): 1789–1858.

Hofmann S.G., Sawyer A.T., Witt A.A. and Oh D. (2010). The effect of mindfulness-based therapy on anxiety and depression: A meta-analytic review. *Journal of Consulting and Clinical Psychology*, 78(2): 169.

Jordan M. and Hinds J. (eds) (2016). *Ecotherapy: Theory, Research & Practice*. London: Palgrave Macmillan.

Kuyken W. et al. (2016). Efficacy of Mindfulness-Based Cognitive Therapy in Prevention of Depressive Relapse: An Individual Patient Data Meta-Analysis from Randomized Trials. *JAMA Psychiatry*, 73(6): 565–574.

McManus S., Bebbington P., Jenkins R. and Brugha T. (eds) (2016). *Mental health and wellbeing in England: Adult Psychiatric Morbidity Survey 2014*. Leeds: NHS Digital.

Mind (2019). Depression. Available at: https://www.Mind.org.uk/information-support/types-of-mental-health-problems/depression/#.Xbgx9dL7RhE

NHS (2019a). Overview – Clinical Depression. Available at: https://www.nhs.uk/mental-health/conditions/clinical-depression/overview/

NHS (2019b). Causes – Clinical Depression. Available at: https://www.nhs.uk/mental-health/conditions/clinical-depression/causes/

NICE (2020). Clinical Knowledge Summaries. Depression – How do I diagnose depression? Available at: https://cks.nice.org.uk/topics/depression/

Parasole R. (2017). The Epidemic of Higher Levels of Depression and Anxiety in Each Successive Generation of Youth: Proposed Causes, Detrimental Effects, and the Introduction of Positive Psychology in the Classroom. *Florida Law Review*, 69(4): 1157–1180.

Sadler K. et al. (2018). Mental Health of Children and Young People in England, 2017: Trends and characteristics. Available at: https://openaccess.city.ac.uk/id/eprint/23650/

Sharma et al. (2016). Suicidality and aggression during antidepressant treatment: systematic review and meta-analyses based on clinical study reports. *BMJ*, 352: i65.

Chapter 4

Postpartum Depression

Aimee Yarrington and Ursula Rolfe

Case study

You are working in an urgent care response car on a Sunday shift in a busy urban centre. At midday you are sent on a referral call for a 32-year-old female patient. There is limited information passed to you about the case, but the caller, who is her husband, is concerned regarding her mental state having found her crying uncontrollably in the bathroom.

On arrival, the husband advises you that she gave birth three weeks ago. He advises that it was a long labour and a forceps birth. She had originally planned on having a home birth but had been transferred to hospital in the first stage of labour as meconium liquor was present and there were concerns about the fetal heart rate. The baby is very unsettled due to reflux, and neither parent has slept well since the birth.

Assessment

- Past medical history: mild asthma not requiring any treatment. Had an uneventful pregnancy.
- Allergies: penicillin.
- Drug history: none.
- Social history: lives with husband in a clean and comfortable house.

On examination

- Appearance: she is still in her nightwear and has not showered or brushed her hair. She is pale and has dark circles below her eyes as if she has not slept all night.
- Behaviour: she is curled up on the bathroom floor crying; however she responds to you and answers all questions appropriately.
- Speech: normal between crying.
- Mood: very low, she says she has been showing little interest in doing anything around the house, but doesn't want to leave it.

- Thought: no formal thought disorders are identified. Form, content and possession appear normal.
- Affect: not applicable.
- Perception: appears normal. She is aware of necessity to provide for the baby and there is no perception that she may cause harm to herself or the baby.
- Cognition: again, appears intact; she is aware of the needs of the baby.
- Insight and judgement: she accepts that it is not right to feel this way in what should be a time of excitement with a new baby. Her husband is asking if she is suffering from postpartum depression, as the health visitor had given him an information leaflet with signs to look out for.
- Risk: she does not state any suicidal thoughts or thoughts of harming the baby.

Clinical observations

- Heart rate: 100 beats/min
- Blood pressure: 110/70 mmHg
- Blood glucose: 4.0 mml/l
- Respiratory rate: 20 breaths/min
- Temperature: 36.7°C
- SpO_2: 95% on room air

Impression

Postpartum depression (PPD), due to the recent birth of a baby and feelings of depression but with cognition and awareness of her need to care for the baby. No suicidal feelings or display of signs of psychosis.

Questions for consideration

- How do you know this patient is suffering PPD?
- Are there differential diagnoses?
- What are some of the challenges in handling this situation and how would you overcome them?
- What advice would you give to the patient?
- How would you manage the situation?

Plan

Specialist input from a perinatal mental health team should be sought. In the interim, a referral for CBT should be made. Self-help strategies should be discussed and also written down as she may not remember all advice given. The risks and benefits of prescribing antidepressants should be discussed with the woman and her husband. As she is breastfeeding, sertraline is the SSRI of choice (NICE, 2018).

Differential diagnoses: depression-related disorders are often hard to distinguish from anxiety, obsessive-compulsive, and trauma-related disorders in the postpartum period and can co-occur with any of these problems. History taking should inquire for symptoms of excessive worry, panic, obsessional thoughts, and compulsive behaviours as well as remote or recent traumatic events associated with nightmares, flashbacks, or other symptoms of post-traumatic stress disorder (PTSD). Family history of depression, bipolar disorder, or postpartum psychosis (PPP) should also be acknowledged if present (Stewart and Vigod, 2019).

Challenges in this situation: women are often reluctant to admit that they have any issues as they do not want to feel like a failure as a mother. There are also challenges in respect to issues around whether she is capable of being able to care for the baby. Ensuring she has additional support from family and friends is important so that she can be kept together with her baby.

Advice given to the patient: self-care is vitally important. Ensuring that she has time to herself to rest, shower and dress will improve her mood. Reassure her that she is doing a good job as a mother and that admission of needing help does not mean she is a failure. Getting out of the house for a walk and gentle exercise will also help to boost her mood. Maintaining a balanced diet will assist in getting the nutrients the body needs and although will not directly influence her depression, it will assist with feeling better. Encourage her not to isolate herself but to find nearby baby groups with mothers who may also be in a similar situation. Isolation is not helpful and talking about feelings has been shown to help new mothers adapt to their new roles within the family unit (Healthline, 2020a).

Aimee Yarrington

Patient voice

'Admitting I was suffering with postpartum depression was the hardest thing I have ever had to do. I did not want family and friends thinking I was a bad mother and didn't love my baby. Having a very intense career, to be suddenly home alone with a newborn was so isolating. I found it easier to just stay in and not venture out. Once I opened up, initially to my husband and then my GP, I found that it was easier to cope with the strategies and personalised plan she advised for me.'

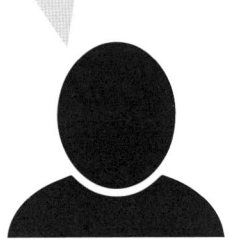

Do not do ...

- Do not assume the patient cannot take care of her baby.

- Do not assume that only women suffer PPD.

- Do not advise her to give up breastfeeding in order to take antidepressant treatments, but discuss the evidence that no medication is licensed for use with breastfeeding. There should be discussions regarding the benefits of breastfeeding over the small amount of medication that is excreted into breast milk.

Recognising postpartum depression

PPD is defined by the Royal College of Psychiatrists (RCPsych, 2019) as a depressive illness, which affects between 10 to 15% of women having a baby. Symptoms are similar to depression and can include low mood, and other symptoms, lasting at least two weeks (RCPsych, 2019). Patients with postpartum depression may struggle to look after themselves and their baby; this is an important factor to consider when it comes to safety-netting. Timing with postpartum depression varies. Often it can present within the first or second month of giving birth; sometimes it can start several months after birth. About a third of women with postpartum depression have symptoms which actually started in pregnancy and continued on after birth (Wisner et al., 2013). PPD should not be confused with the baby blues. A recognized condition that can affect up to 80% of new mothers in the first few days after birth (NCT, 2018). This is mainly due to the regulation of hormones after birth. Symptoms include heightened emotions, tearfulness without reason, anxiety and feelings of being overwhelmed (NCT, 2018). When these symptoms present after the first few days and last more than 10-14 days the diagnosis of PPD is more likely (NHS, 2018a).

PPD is not exclusive to women as it can affect partners too (Pras Ramluggun et al., 2020). The transition into parenthood often affects both partners and although the cases of female PPD are discussed and are the main content of this chapter, it should not be forgotten that partners can also suffer from PPD and should be treated and managed accordingly. There is evidence to suggest that untreated partner depression can cause emotional and behavioural problems in their children and is more prevalent in male infants (Kvalevaag et al., 2013).

Understanding the condition

There are different theories about the causes of postpartum depression. However, some patients will be more at risk of developing postpartum depression if they have had (Mind, 2019):

- Previous mental health problems

- There are biological causes (for example, hormonal changes)

- Lack of support

- Difficult childhood experiences

- Previous or current abuse (for example domestic violence, verbal and/or emotional abuse, sexual assault or financial abuse)

- Low self-esteem

- Stressful living conditions (for example poverty, poor housing, insecure employment)

- Major life events (e.g. major illness or death, relationship break-up, moving house or loss of their job).

Several studies have found a significant association between the woman's birthing experiences and what is viewed as a negative experience, can also be a contributing factor in the woman developing PPD (Bell and Anderson, 2016).

There are several misconceptions regarding PPD, one being that it will go away by itself, but also that it is less severe than other types of depression, that it is entirely due to hormonal changes, that it is different from depression present before childbirth and that there is no risk of recurrence in the non-postpartum period (National Collaborating Centre for Mental Health, 2014).

Self-help ideas for your patient

Experiencing PPD can be very distressing for your patient, and they may be struggling to reach out or communicate. It is therefore noteworthy that you can start your care of this patient with some supportive ideas to encourage their engagement in their condition. There are some tips you can suggest as well as some supportive tools which may help your patient reach out to others.

Importance of physical wellbeing

Can your patient get out of the house for a walk or even just a change of scenery? Even if it's only for 10 minutes or so. Encourage her to keep active as gentle activity is not only good for her, but it can also enhance her mood. Does she have any family or friends she could rely on to help out for a few minutes a day while she has a shower, or even someone to have a cup of tea with and an adult conversation. These activities may help to improve and lift her mood (Mind, 2019; NHS, 2018b).

As well as exercise, nutrition is also important. Ask your patient about her diet as a poor diet can often lead to a low mood and lack of energy. With a newborn in the house, meal planning in advance and using foods that are easy to prepare by batch cooking can be a positive way forward for your patient. When she doesn't feel well or feels low on energy, it means that there will be access to quick foods and she can therefore maintain a healthy and nutritious diet even when she doesn't feel up to cooking (Mind, 2019; NHS, 2018b). Another aspect new mothers struggle with is getting used to sleep deprivation. There is a certain level of expectation of sleep deprivation as a baby's sleep pattern is often erratic and this is normal. However, poor sleep has a direct relationship with poor mental health (Tham et al., 2016; Park et al., 2013). The phrase 'sleep when your baby sleeps' is always advised; however, with babies that don't sleep well, this is often difficult. If possible, finding a friend to mind the baby or taking it in turns with a partner overnight can often help with sleep deprivation (Mind, 2019; NHS, 2018c). This may be difficult for those who are isolated or solo parenting.

Reaching out to others

Ask your patient if she is attending any activities with her baby; local mother and baby groups are often a source of support for mothers who may be in a similar situation. Reaching out to others may be the last thing your patient wants to do but there are several online forums which provide support and enable access to other mums who are not in the direct vicinity, for example, Mumsnet or Netmums. Pandas (www. pandasfoundation.org.uk) also provides support on the phone or in groups specifically tailored towards antenatal and postpartum support. It's good to be aware, however, that there are also some negative aspects to accessing social media, many portray a rosy glow to parenthood and only recognized support groups should be recommended.

Reflective practices for your patient

Considering personal needs when your patient is a mother to a newborn is difficult. She may often forget to perform basic personal hygiene. Inform her that little things like getting washed and dressed can make a big difference to her mood. Getting into a routine with her baby will also provide structure for the day. It may feel very overwhelming and difficult with a newborn and she may feel she has no time for herself. Taking a small amount of time, perhaps even just five minutes to herself to recharge and unwind is very important (Mind, 2019; NHS, 2018b).

Clinical treatment and management

The treatment of PPD is extremely important because not only does this impact on the woman's quality of life, but also on family life. A very large study of almost 10,000 women with various levels of PPD found that the children of the women whose PPD persisted were more likely to develop behavioural problems as well as lower grades of attainment (Netsi et al., 2018). There are several options in regard to treatment for PPD, but before starting or altering treatment, discussions should, ideally, take place with a perinatal mental health specialist. All treatment options should be on an individual basis, there are, as with all mental health conditions, no blanket care options. Treatment options should be made in conjunction with your patient and her past mental health history should be taken into consideration. Also consider the relationships with and the level of support she has from her family or carers and the needs of her family, for example, other children (NICE, 2018).

NICE (2018) also suggests first discussing concerns your patient has about her baby including her plans around breastfeeding and the possible risks associated with taking medication when breastfeeding. It is also important to consider and discuss the risks and potential harm of stopping medication such as antidepressants abruptly or changing treatment. Then there is the risk of not treating depression which also requires careful consideration. There are several treatment options recommended by NICE (2018). Discuss the potential benefits of each treatment and remember to consider treatment options that would enable your patient to breastfeed if she wishes to do so. They include: psychological treatment or talking therapies, antidepressant treatment or a combination of both (Table 4.1).

Table 4.1 Treatment options for PPD

Severity of PPD	Treatment options
All PPD	• Self-care strategies • Sleep protection • Exercise • Investigate and manage social stressors as well as medical and psychiatric co-morbidities
Mild to moderate PPD (or PPD not in remission from self-care and psychological strategies)	• Psychological treatments, including CBT and IPT. • Add SSRI if insufficient response (consider lactation safety)
Severe PPD	• SSRI alone (consider lactation safety) or with psychological intervention • Consider antidepressant switch if no response to SSRI alone.

Source: Adapted from Stewart and Vigod (2019).

Psychological treatment

Psychological treatment includes cognitive behavioural therapy (CBT), which aims to help your patient understand her behaviours and thoughts. CBT is available on the NHS for patients with depression as mentioned in the previous chapter. Interpersonal therapy (IPT) is another type of therapy that focuses on your patient and her relationships with other people; it is based on the idea that personal relationships are at the centre of psychological issues. Several studies have found that IPT may be as effective as antidepressants for treating depression (Healthline, 2020b). Both CBT and IPT are short-term therapy options and are often used for the less severe cases of PPD. In a recent narrative review, Stamou, García-Palacios and Botella (2018) add that CBT can be effective in the short term or up to six months later; interestingly CBT using virtual reality has never been used for the treatment of PPD.

Medication

Before considering antidepressant medications, NICE (2018) recommend that paramedics refer to or contact specialist advice, ideally from a specialist perinatal mental health team or from secondary psychiatric care. Medication choices are often dependent on your patient's method of feeding. For a patient with a history of severe depression who initially presents with mild depression in the postpartum period, consider a tricyclic antidepressant (TCA), selective serotonin reuptake inhibitor (SSRI), or serotonin-noradrenaline reuptake inhibitor (SNRI). The choice of medication should also be based on her previous response to medication and the risk profile for her and her baby (NICE, 2018). For patients who are breastfeeding, reassurance regarding medication may be found on the Breastfeeding Network website. They recommend that sertraline be the antidepressant of choice due to its short half-life and low likelihood of accumulation in the infant (Jones, 2021). The lowest effective dose should be prescribed, but ensuring that the depression is still adequately treated (NICE, 2018). Many patients will want to avoid TCAs due to possible side effects causing sleepiness (Jones, 2021). When considering which antidepressant to prescribe for patients who are breastfeeding, seek specialist advice and also discuss this with a paediatrician if the baby was premature or has health problems. NICE (2018) advise clinicians to consider the benefits of breastfeeding for both the patient and her baby. At time of publication, it should be noted that there is limited research and uncertainty about the safety of these medications for the breastfeeding baby and the potential risks associated to both mother and baby. Also consider the risks linked to switching from, or stopping, a previously effective medication.

Safeguarding

If your patient does not want to be treated, they should be counselled about the potential consequences of not having treatment for PPD. According to NICE (2018) there is some evidence to suggest there is a risk of harm to both the patient and her baby including an increase in sudden infant death syndrome (SIDS) and self-harm. The most common treatment options encompass a combination of all treatment options, along with the self-help options discussed above (p. 61).

According to NICE (2018), if your patient requires admission for a mental health problem within 12 months of childbirth, they should be admitted to a specialist mother and baby unit, unless there are specific reasons for not doing so. Admission of babies to general psychiatric wards is not advised. Refer your patient to a secondary mental health service, ideally a specialist perinatal mental health service, for immediate assessment, that is, within 4 hours of referral, if she has a sudden onset of symptoms suggestive of postpartum psychosis. According to the NHS (2020) postpartum psychosis is characterised by:

- Hallucinations
- Delusions
- Manic mood
- Low mood
- Loss of inhibitions
- Feeling suspicious or fearful
- Restlessness

- Feeling very confused

- Behaving in a way that is out of character.

Consider urgently referring to a secondary mental health team (preferably with a special interest in perinatal mental health) if your patient presents with the following (NICE, 2018):

- Is severely depressed and presents a considerable immediate risk of harm to herself or other people – admission may be required if clinically indicated.

- Shows evidence of severe self-neglect or is unable to care for her infant.

- Has a possible diagnosis of bipolar disorder. See Chapter 9 – Bipolar Disorder (p. 115) for more detail.

- Has a history of severe mental ill-health, including postpartum depression, puerperal psychosis, or bipolar disorder (during pregnancy or the postpartum period or at any other time).

Refer your patient to a specialist substance misuse service if, in addition to depression, she has harmful or dependent drug or alcohol misuse in pregnancy or the postpartum period. Refer or seek specialist advice if your patient is considering starting, stopping, or switching antidepressant treatment and if she is not responding to treatment appropriate to the severity of her depression. NICE (2018) adds that specialist advice may be sought ideally from a specialist perinatal mental health team where available, or from a secondary mental health service.

To conclude, NICE (2018) advises you to consider the following additional factors when deciding whether to refer or seek specialist advice: your patient's preference, her past medical history and response to treatment/s, her degree of functional impairment and whether she has significant co-morbidities or specific symptoms that increase her risk factors.

References

Bell A.F. and Andersson E. (2016). The birth experience and women's postnatal depression: A systematic review. *Midwifery*, 39: 112–123.

Healthline (2020a). 7 Ways to Cope with Postpartum Depression. Available at: https://www.healthline.com/health/depression/how-to-deal-with-postpartum-depression

Healthline (2020b). Interpersonal Therapy. Available at: https://www.healthline.com/health/depression/interpersonal-therapy

Jones W. (2021). Antidepressants and Breastfeeding. *The Breastfeeding Network*. Available at: https://www.breastfeedingnetwork.org.uk/antidepressants/

Kvalevaag A.L. et al. (2013). Paternal Mental Health and Socioemotional and Behavioral Development in Their Children. *Pediatrics*, 131(2): e463–469.

Mind (2019). Postnatal depression and perinatal mental health. What causes perinatal mental health problems? Available at: https://www.Mind.org.uk/information-support/types-of-mental-health-problems/postnatal-depression-and-perinatal-mental-health/causes/#.XfJhotL7RhE

National Collaborating Centre for Mental Health (2014). Antenatal and postnatal mental health. The NICE guideline on clinical management and service guidance (updated edition). The British Psychological Society and the Royal College of Psychiatrists. Available at https://www.nice.org.uk/guidance/cg192/evidence/full-guideline-pdf-4840896925

Netsi E. et al. (2018). Association of Persistent and Severe Postnatal Depression With Child Outcomes. *JAMA Psychiatry*, 75(3): 247–253.

NCT (2018). The Baby blues: what to expect (online). Available at: https://www.nct.org.uk/life-parent/how-you-might-be-feeling/baby-blues-what-expect

NHS (2018a). Feeling depressed after childbirth: The baby blues. (online) Available at: https://www.nhs.uk/conditions/baby/support-and-services/feeling-depressed-after-childbirth/

NHS (2018b). Overview – Postnatal depression. Available at: https://www.nhs.uk/conditions/post-natal-depression/

NHS (2018c). Helping your baby to sleep. Available at: https://www.nhs.uk/conditions/pregnancy-and-baby/getting-baby-to-sleep/

NHS (2019). Overview – Cognitive behavioural therapy (CBT). Available at: https://www.nhs.uk/mental-health/talking-therapies-medicine-treatments/talking-therapies-and-counselling/cognitive-behavioural-therapy-cbt/overview/

NHS (2020). Postpartum psychosis. Available at: https://www.nhs.uk/conditions/post-partum-psychosis/

NICE (2018). Clinical Knowledge Summaries. Depression – antenatal and postnatal. Available at: https://cks.nice.org.uk/topics/depression-antenatal-postnatal/

NICE (2020). Depression – antenatal and postnatal. Available at https://cks.nice.org.uk/topics/depression-antenatal-postnatal

Park E.M., Meltzer-Brody S. and Stickgold R. (2013). Poor sleep maintenance and subjective sleep quality are associated with postpartum maternal depression symptom severity. *Archives of Women's Mental Health*, 16(6): 539–547.

Ramluggun P., Kamara A. and Anjoyeb M. (2020) Postnatal depression in fathers: a quiet struggle? *British Journal of Mental Health Nursing*, 9(4): 1–8.

Royal College of Psychiatrists (2019). Postnatal depression. Available at: https://www.rcpsych.ac.uk/mental-health/problems-disorders/post-natal-depression

Stamou G., García-Palacios A. and Botella C. (2018). Cognitive-Behavioural therapy and interpersonal psychotherapy for the treatment of post-natal depression: a narrative review. *BMC Psychology*, 6(28).

Stewart D.E. and Vigod S.N. (2019). Postpartum Depression: Pathophysiology, Treatment, and Emerging Therapeutics. *Annual Review of Medicine*, 70: 183–196.

Tham E.K.H. et al. (2016). Associations between poor subjective prenatal sleep quality and postnatal depression and anxiety symptoms. *Journal of Affective Disorders*, 202: 91–94.

Wisner K. et al. (2013). Onset Timing, Thoughts of Self-harm, and Diagnoses in Postpartum Women with Screen-positive Depression Findings. *JAMA Psychiatry*, 70(5): 490–498.

Anxiety Disorders

Ursula Rolfe

Case study

You are working the last of your run of day shifts on a double-crewed ambulance in a busy inner-city location. While trying to grab a quick coffee at the local café, your radio beeps just as you're about to order. You crawl through the traffic to reach Martin, a 52-year-old male who feels like he can't catch his breath.

Martin tells you that he began to feel breathless after speaking to his daughter who has recently moved away to study at university. He says he is extremely anxious about her but has been trying to hold in his emotions so as not to cause any worry. As well as feeling breathless, Martin has also been feeling restless and has difficulty concentrating. This is not the first time the symptoms have been felt and they are subsiding as you are talking to him.

Assessment

- Past medical history: generalised anxiety disorder (GAD), hypertension.
- Drug history: escitalopram (10 milligrams daily), ramipril (2.5 milligrams daily).
- Allergies: no known drug allergies.
- Social history: lives with his wife. Independent with no care needs. Works in office environment. Non-smoker. Drinks socially – approximately 6 units a week. No illicit drug use.

On examination

- Appearance: clean, well-kept and dressed appropriately for the environment. No evidence of self-harm.
- Behaviour: clearly anxious but maintaining eye contact and behaving appropriately.
- Speech: answering questions and conversing appropriately and coherently.

- Mood: expresses worry about his daughter and also other aspects of life but does not demonstrate signs of depression.
- Affect: generally anxious, but becomes flat and sad at times when discussing daughter.
- Thoughts: generally anxious but able to rationalise thoughts. No thoughts of self-harm or suicide.
- Perception: no abnormal perceptions.
- Cognition: orientated to time, place and person. Able to process and recall information freely.
- Insight and judgement: understands current presentation is linked to diagnosis of GAD and wants further help.
- Risk: No previous history or apparent risk to self or others.

Clinical observations

- Heart rate: 90 beats/min
- Blood pressure: 144/88 mmHg
- Blood glucose: 5.1 mml/l
- Respiratory rate: 16 breaths/min
- Temperature: 36.7°C
- SpO_2: 98% on room air

Cardiovascular and respiratory assessments do not suggest a physical cause for Martin's symptoms.

Impression

1. Anxiety/panic attack
2. GAD

Questions for Consideration

1. How do you know that this patient is experiencing an anxiety/panic attack and GAD? Are there any other potential diagnoses?
2. Where is the most appropriate place for this patient to receive help and support?
3. What advice would you give to this patient? How would you ensure the patient's GP is aware of the consultation.

Plan

GAD is a common condition affecting approximately 5% of the adult population in the UK. Symptoms may present both physically and psychologically including the familiar symptoms of anxiety or panic attack. There is no immediate need for Martin to go to hospital and various community treatment options are available. A Selective Serotonin Reuptake Inhibitor (SSRI) has already been prescribed, but arranging a review with the patient's GP to discuss an increase in dose or medication change would be beneficial. It would be appropriate for the patient to arrange this themselves if they feel comfortable speaking to their GP. Talking therapies, relaxation techniques and Cognitive Behavioural Therapy (CBT) may also be useful as an alternative or in conjunction with pharmacological treatments. Taking a calm and reassuring approach to Martin is likely to be all that is needed in the pre-hospital setting after potential physical causes have been excluded. Having an awareness and signposting to relevant information websites (such as www.nhs.uk) and local self-referral services will also allow you to offer something practical before other treatment options can be arranged.

Andrew Hichisson

Patient voice

'My anxiety and how it manifests isn't just a way for me to get attention, I am not pretending.'

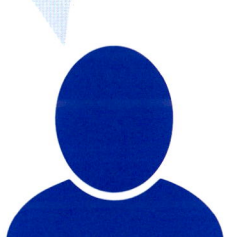

Do not do …

- Be aware that in a minority of people aged under 30 years of age, SSRIs and SNRIs are associated with an increased risk of suicidal thinking and self-harm (NICE, 2017).

- Although you need to get a good medical history, try not to bring up the word anxiety too much; rephrase things and ask about symptoms.

- Don't expect your patient to have immediate relief from his disorder because controlling anxiety takes time.

- Try not to enable your patient's anxieties.

Recognising anxiety

Anxiety is defined as 'a feeling people get in a situation that is threatening or difficult' (RCPsych, 2019). The feelings of anxiety stop when the patient gets accustomed to the situation, leaves it, or it changes. Anxiety can be experienced in many different ways and this chapter will consider some of the most commonly diagnosed anxiety disorders. These include generalised anxiety disorder (GAD), social anxiety disorder, panic disorder and phobias.

GAD refers to patients having regular and uncontrollable worries about a variety of things in their daily lives. This is quite a broad consideration and should be diagnosed by an appropriate GP or mental health specialist. Up to 5% of the UK population are diagnosed with GAD. It affects more women than men and is most common between the ages of 35–59 according to the NHS (2020). The differential diagnosis of anxiety disorders include major depression, somatic symptoms disorders as well as physical illnesses such as coronary heart or lung diseases and others (Bandelow, Michaelis and Wedekind, 2017).

Social anxiety disorder refers to patients who experience extreme fear or anxiety triggered by parties, workplaces or situations where people will be required to communicate with another person.

Panic disorder is recognised by frequent panic attacks without a clear cause or trigger (Mind, 2021). Patients will feel constantly afraid of experiencing another panic attack which could itself trigger another. Phobias are described as an extreme fear or anxiety triggered by certain situations (e.g. social situations/flying/blood) or certain objects (e.g. spiders). Evidence suggests that rates of misdiagnosis or missed diagnoses for GAD and panic disorders remain high as symptoms are often ascribed to physical causes (Locke, Kirst and Schultz, 2015).

Other sources also include post-traumatic stress disorder (PTSD) and obsessive-compulsive disorder (OCD), but these conditions will be considered separately in later chapters of the book.

Occasional anxiety is part of life but people with anxiety disorders experience anxiety that does not go away and may worsen over time. Symptoms can interfere with daily activities such as working life and impact on relationships.

Understanding anxiety

Feeling anxious elicits different feelings and has physiological effects on the body. These effects can include (Mind, 2021):

- A churning feeling in the stomach
- Feeling light-headed or dizzy

- Pins and needles
- Feeling restless
- Headaches or other aches and pains
- Tachypnoea
- Tachycardia
- Sweating or hot flushes
- Problems sleeping
- Bruxism (teeth grinding)
- Nausea
- Changes in sex drive
- Panic attacks.

The following causes can contribute to anxiety disorders (RCPsych, 2019):

- Genes
- Trauma
- Drugs
- Mental health problems
- Physical health problems
- A combination of the above.

It has been suggested that some people are born anxious and that research suggests it could be inherited via genes (Morris-Rosendahl, 2002; Gottschalk and Domschke, 2017). Past trauma or negative childhood experiences are a common cause of anxiety as are experiences such as physical or emotional abuse, neglect, losing a parent and being bullied or socially excluded. Drugs and medication can sometimes induce anxiety as a side effect.

Patients with other mental health problems, such as depression, often also experience anxiety. Physical problems such as living with a serious, ongoing or life-threatening physical health condition may cause anxiety (Mind, 2021).

Diagnosis of anxiety disorders is not simple but diagnostic criteria are usually reflected in the *DSM-5* (American Psychiatric Association, 2013). According to Bystritsky et al. (2013) many people presenting with anxiety have co-morbidities. For example, in some patients with GAD and social anxiety disorders the presence of co-morbidities is a rule rather than an exception (Bystritsky et al., 2013).

The most common anxiety disorder – GAD – should be suspected in a person who reports chronic, excessive worry not related to particular circumstances and symptoms such as restlessness, insomnia and muscle tension (NICE, 2017). As previously mentioned, the *DSM-5* criteria include: at least six months of excessive, difficult to control worry about everyday issues, that is disproportionate to any inherent risk, and causes distress or impairment; the worry is not confined to features of another mental disorder, or as a result of substance abuse, or a general medical condition; the person experiences at least 3 of the following symptoms most of the time: restlessness/ nervousness, being easily fatigued, poor concentration, irritability, muscle tension, or sleep disturbance (American Psychiatric Association, 2013). Interestingly, in primary care, people with GAD often present with physical symptoms such as headaches, muscle tension, gastrointestinal symptoms, back pain, insomnia and may not easily report worry or distress (NICE, 2017). Also be aware that the following factors increase the likelihood of a GAD diagnosis; when the patient:

- Is female with a family history of anxiety and/or other anxiety disorders

- Is under emotional or physical stress

- Has a history of physical or emotional trauma

- Experiences persistent pain or physical illness

- Has a history of substance abuse

- Makes repeated visits with the same physical symptoms that have not responded to treatment (such as insomnia, fatigue or headaches).

It would be prudent to carry out a physical examination as your patient may be exhibiting tachycardia, tachypnoea, trembling and an exaggerated startle response. The GAD questionnaire referred to as the GAD-7 is an assessment tool used to determine the severity of GAD. NICE (2017) advises clinicians to consider differential diagnoses, which may include: situational anxiety, adjustment disorder, depression, panic disorder, social phobia, OCD, PTSD and others. You are not required to newly diagnose patients you suspect may have an anxiety disorder.

Self-help ideas for your patient

Living with anxiety can be hard for your patient but there are supportive measures you can suggest to your patients that might help them. It is therefore noteworthy that you can start your care of this patient with some supportive ideas to encourage their engagement in their condition. There are some tips you can suggest as well as some supportive tools which may help your patient reach out to others.

Importance of physical wellbeing

We underestimate how exercise, diet and sleep can impact physical health. Exercise is helpful for managing stress and anxiety. Mind (2020) suggests also encouraging your patient to get enough sleep. Lack of sleep often increases feelings of anxiety. Eating regular, healthy meals can contribute to improving mood and energy levels.

Breathing exercises can help with managing anxiety and feeling more in control. There is also supporting evidence according to Mind (2020) that mindfulness (giving your full attention to the moment) helps reduce anxiety. Interestingly, NICE (2017) adds that mindfulness is not helpful for social anxiety. Mindfulness tends to work for some people while others say it makes their anxiety worse. Support your patient in making an individual choice that suits them.

A systematic review by Jayakody, Gunadasa and Hosker (2014) noted that exercise seems to be effective as an adjunct treatment for anxiety disorders but cautioned that this was less effective compared with treatment with antidepressants. It was also noted that exercise also appeared to reduce anxiety symptoms.

Reaching out to others

Although talking to others may be difficult for those who have anxiety, it may provide some relief. Suggest a friend or relative whom your patient trusts. There are a variety of charities and organisations available to consult, for example, the Samaritans and Anxiety UK; these organisations provide helplines which are easily accessible.

Peer support brings people who have similar experiences together and there are many organisations such as Anxiety UK, No More Panic, Triumph over Phobia and Anxiety Care which run support groups, forums and helplines via their websites. However, Lloyd Evans, Mayo-Wilson and Harrison (2014) advise caution, as their systematic review and meta-analysis demonstrates that current evidence does not support mandatory peer support programmes, especially for those with severe mental health illness. This should be considered as an adjunct.

Reflective practices for your patient

Often patients will feel like they cannot control their worries. Some will feel that continuing to worry feels useful or that something negative will happen if they stop worrying. There are different ways of addressing these worries. You could advise your patient to set aside specific time to focus on their worries; this will help reassure your patient that they haven't forgotten their worry (Mind, 2020). You could also suggest that your patient writes down their worries and keeps them in a safe place. Keeping a diary might be useful as it can help patients spot patterns in what triggers their anxiety or identify the early signs. They could also write down what is going well.

Clinical treatment and management

Anxiety disorders in general are treated with psychotherapy, medication or a combination of both (NIMH, 2019). Advise your patient to consult their GP for the most suitable treatment and management plan. You can, however, explain some of the treatments the patient can expect in more detail.

Psychotherapy, also known as 'talk therapy', can help with anxiety disorders but it needs to be directed to the patient's specific anxieties (NIMH, 2019). A popular talking therapy is cognitive behavioural therapy (CBT), which teaches patients different ways of behaving, thinking and reacting to situations or feelings that cause anxiety. It can also aid in learning and practising social skills which are necessary for treating social anxiety disorder (NIMH, 2019). CBT can be conducted in groups or during one-to-one sessions and patients are often given 'homework' to complete between sessions. In a recent study by Gallagher et al. (2020), it was found that CBT strongly increased different domains of wellbeing, and increases in wellbeing during treatment appear to be strongly linked with anxiety symptom reduction.

It's important to remind your patient that medication will not cure their anxiety disorder but it will help relieve its associated symptoms. The most common medication used for anxiety disorders are anti-anxiety drugs such as antidepressants, benzodiazepines and beta-blockers (NICE, 2017). According to Bandelow, Michaelis and Wedekind (2017), in most cases, drug treatment and CBT may substantially improve the quality of life in those with GAD.

NICE (2017) recommends a stepped approach to managing GAD:

Step 1 is to assess the severity of GAD. NICE (2017) suggests using the GAD-7 questionnaire as a validated assessment tool. This may be found on the NICE website. Also ask your patient about factors that may affect the course, development and severity of GAD; these include co-morbidities such as depression or other medical conditions, substance abuse, and environmental stressors, such as financial worries, or poor interpersonal relationships. Always consider your patient's risk of suicide. Refer your patient to information leaflets or materials about GAD and arrange for active monitoring of the patient's symptoms and function. You will not be able to actively monitor in the pre-hospital environment, but you can advise the patient that this is what they can expect in primary care. You can, alternatively, refer them to their locally appropriate healthcare professional who is able to initiate treatment for them following a full risk assessment.

Step 2 is for patients who are not improving following Step 1 intervention. NICE (2017) recommends that these patients need to be referred for low intensity psychological interventions-based CBT.

Step 3 is appropriate for patients who have marked functional impairment or GAD that has not improved following Step 2 interventions. NICE (2017) recommends that Step 3 include high intensity psychological intervention such as CBT *or* drug treatment. The choice between psychological intervention and drug treatment should be patient led as there is no evidence to suggest one is more effective than the other.

The first line of drug treatment is usually the selective serotonin reuptake inhibitor (SSRI) (NICE, 2017). Please note, in a minority of people aged under 30 years of age, SSRIs and SNRIs are associated with an increased risk of suicidal thinking and self-harm (NICE, 2017). Anyone in this age group should therefore be seen within one week of the SSRI first being prescribed and the risk of suicidal thinking and self-harm should be monitored weekly for the first month of treatment. A systematic review looking at the efficacy of SSRIs and SNRIs add that higher doses of SSRIs within the therapeutic range are associated with greater treatment benefits; however, higher doses of SNRIs are not (Jakubovski et al., 2017).

NICE (2017) adds that benzodiazepines should not be offered to the patient for the treatment of GAD; also, if you work in a primary care environment, do not prescribe an antipsychotic to your patient for the treatment of GAD.

Step 4 is for patients with severe anxiety and what NICE (2017) terms as marked functional impairment, and/or GAD that has not improved following Step 3 interventions. These patients should be referred for specialist treatment which can include complex drug and/or psychological interventions, possibly administered on an inpatient basis or with the support of multiple agencies. These patients are often at risk of self-harm, self-neglect or present with a substantial co-morbidity such as personality disorder, substance abuse or complex physical health issues. NICE (2017) advises that some of these patients may also be at risk of suicide and should have a same-day referral to the crisis resolution and home treatment team.

For all patients with GAD who are managed in primary care, NICE (2017) also advises that self-care advice relating to sleep and exercise should be offered to the patient – as discussed in the self-care section of this chapter. Talk to your patient about sleep hygiene. This includes going to bed and waking up at the same time every day. Advise them to stop drinking alcohol after 18.00 hours and to avoid caffeine after 15.00 hours. Suggest to your patient that if they cannot sleep, they should get out of bed to avoid negative associations with sleeping. Talking about the importance of exercise is appropriate as well. As discussed above, regular exercise can improve overall health and has shown to improve anxiety symptoms.

How should you assess a patient you believe is a suicide risk?

As with all mental health issues, safeguarding is essential as well as risk assessment. To assess your patient's suicide risk, you need to determine whether they feel hopeless or that life is not worth living. NICE (2017) recommends that you do not avoid using the word 'suicide'. They suggest asking some of the following questions to your patient:

- Do you ever think about suicide?
- Have you made any plans for ending your life?
- Do you have the means for doing this available to you?
- What has kept you from acting on these thoughts?

It is important to follow up on 'not really' answers. You can also use the IPAP tool to help guide your risk assessment, which can be found in Chapter 2 – Decision Making (p. 25).

NICE (2017) also suggests that patients require regular reassessment of the risk of suicide throughout their course of treatment, if this is something you are able to provide in your area of practice. Also be aware of what NICE defines as 'danger periods', for example, when initiating treatment, changes in treatment, or at times of increased personal stress.

NICE (2017) has identified risk factors that increase the risk of suicide including:

- Previous attempts at suicide or self-harm
- Family history of suicide
- Feeling hopeless
- Being male and under the age of 30
- Advanced age
- Single or living alone
- History of substance or alcohol abuse
- A diagnosis of psychosis
- Recent initiation of antidepressants
- History of anxiety, panic attacks and agitation
- Concurrent physical illness and severe depression.

Also consider assessing the adequacy of social support and current personal circumstances of each patient. NICE (2017) also suggests identifying factors that could reduce the risk of suicide, including good social support and responsibility for children.

References

American Psychiatric Association (2013). *Diagnostic and Statistical Manual of Mental Disorders (DSM-5), Fifth Edition*. Washington, DC: American Psychiatric Association Publishing, 87–120.

Bandelow B., Michaelis S. and Wedekind D. (2017). Treatment of anxiety disorders. *Dialogues in Clinical Neuroscience*, 19(2): 93–107.

Bystritsky A., Khalsa S.S., Cameron M.E. and Schiffman J. (2013). Current diagnosis and treatment of anxiety disorders. *Pharmacy and Therapeutics Journal*, 38(1): 30–57.

Gallagher M.W. et al. (2020). Trajectories of change in well-being during cognitive behavioural therapies for anxiety disorders: Quantifying the impact and covariation with improvements in anxiety. *American Psychological Association*, 57(3): 379–390.

Gottschalk M.G. and Domschke K. (2017). Genetics of generalized anxiety disorder and related traits. *Dialogues in Clinical Neuroscience*, 19(2): 159–168.

Jakubovski E. et al. (2017). Systematic review and meta-analysis: Dose-response curve of SSRIs and SNRIs in anxiety disorders. *Depression and Anxiety*, 36(3): 198–212.

Jayakody K., Gunadasa S. and Hosker C. (2014). Exercise for anxiety disorders: systematic review. *British Journal of Sports Medicine*, 48: 187–196.

Lloyd-Evans B., Mayo-Wilson E. and Harrison B. (2014). A systematic review and meta-analysis of randomised controlled trials of peer support for people with severe mental illness. *BMC Psychiatry*, 14(39): 1–12.

Locke A., Kirst N. and Shultz C. (2015). Diagnosis and management of generalized anxiety disorder and panic disorder in adults. *American Family Physician*, 91(9): 617–624.

Mind (2021). Anxiety and panic attacks. Available at: https://www.mind.org.uk/information-support/types-of-mental-health-problems/anxiety-and-panic-attacks/about-anxiety/disorders

Morris-Rosendahl D.J. (2002). Are there anxious genes? *Dialogues in Clinical Neuroscience*, 4(3): 251–260.

National Institute of Mental Health (2019). Anxiety Disorders. Available at: https://www.nimh.nih.gov/health/topics/anxiety-disorders/index.shtml

NHS (2020). Overview: Generalised anxiety disorder in adults. Available at: https://www.nhs.uk/conditions/generalised-anxiety-disorder/

NICE (2017). Clinical Knowledge Summaries. Generalised anxiety disorder. Available at: https://cks.nice.org.uk/topics/generalized-anxiety-disorder/

NICE (2019). Generalised anxiety disorder and panic disorder in adults: management. Clinical guideline [CG113]. Available at: https://www.nice.org.uk/guidance/CG113

Royal College of Psychiatrists (2019). Anxiety, panic and phobias. Available at: https://www.rcpsych.ac.uk/mental-health/problems-disorders/anxiety-panic-and-phobias?searchTerms=anxiety

Obsessive-Compulsive Disorder

Chapter 6

Ursula Rolfe

Case study

It is Monday afternoon and you are working on a double-crewed ambulance with your regular crew mate. You are dispatched to a local university hall of residence for a 19-year-old male with breathing difficulties. On arrival you are met by a flatmate who tells you that you are here to see Jack who is struggling to breathe.

On entering the flat, you find 'Jack' in his room in a highly distressed state, anxious in the midst of what you quickly recognise as a panic attack. With reassurance and breathing coaching Jack begins to calm and allows you to take a full set of physical observations, all of which are now within normal parameters. Jack says that he has always been easily stressed and anxious but has sought no help for this before.

After Jack has become calm and you have explained what has happened, he tells you that he is worried that he is 'having a breakdown'. He explains that he is having thoughts that something terrible is going to happen to him and that someone is going to break into his room and steal his laptop and as a consequence he will be kicked off his course for failing to complete an assignment. He says 'I know it's ridiculous if I think about it' but that recently he has been repeatedly checking his door is locked up to 100 times. This has been impacting on his progress with his course as he is skipping lectures, having to return home multiple times on the way to university or leaving within 10 minutes of arrival to go home to check his door is locked. Jack tells you he feels as if he is not in control of his thoughts but is aware that they are not founded in truth and that if he doesn't act on them he becomes so anxious as to induce a panic attack.

Assessment

- Past medical history: Jack has no pre-morbid physical illness.
- Allergies: none.
- Drug history: none.
- Social history: university student.

On examination

- Appearance: appropriately dressed with good personal hygiene. No evidence of any wounds or injuries.
- Behaviour: initially restless and very anxious, rapid shallow breathing, wringing hands and pacing around his room in keeping with psychomotor agitation. Following a period of reassurance and breathing coaching he is able to sit and converse. No hostility or irritability. Good rapport established.
- Speech: normal rate, rhythm and flow with no poverty of speech or disinhibition.
- Mood: reports ongoing low mood and rates mood as generally 3/10 with 0 as lowest. Denies diurnal mood variation. Finds his anxieties and intrusive thoughts impact on his mood causing him to feel low. Not labile in mood, reported or observed.
- Thoughts: intrusive thoughts that his room is not secure. Catastrophising of potential consequences. Good insight and thoughts in keeping with intrusive thoughts rather than delusional belief structure.
- Perception: denies hallucinations of all modalities. Not observed to be distracted or responding to apparent psychotic stimuli.
- Affect: appropriate reactive affect with no evidence of blunting, mask-like affect or labile.
- Cognition: no apparent impairment.
- Insight and judgement: good insight into his mental health. Able to identify that he is prone to anxiety and how this affects his mood. Understands that the thoughts are irrational but continues to act on them. He is insightful that he is struggling with his mental health and wants help to return to his normal self.
- Risk: no history of risk to self or others. Denies any thoughts of harming self or others. Longer-term risk of issues with university as currently impairing his ability to engage/attend lectures.

Clinical observations

- Heart rate: 76 beats/min
- Blood pressure: 129/84 mmHg
- Blood glucose: 5.9 mml/l
- Respiratory rate: 17 breaths/min
- Temperature: 36.5°C
- SpO_2: 98% on room air

Impression

Panic attack secondary to obsessive-compulsive disorder (OCD)

Questions for consideration

- Which elements of the assessment are more specific to OCD?
- Who could you speak to for further advice/management plans?
- Where could you direct Jack for assistance? (e.g. student support services)

Plan

Following discussion with Jack he says he doesn't want to go to the emergency department (ED) as he thinks he will find it too stressful and he will just leave to come home and check his flat. As there is no immediate risk to himself or others, you agree that ED is probably not the best option and with Jack's consent, you liaise with his GP to book an urgent appointment to discuss his mental health. Jack's GP agrees with your working impression and suggests that she will speak to Jack about the options available including psychological therapies such as Cognitive Behavioural Therapy (CBT) and the potential need for medication. You also encourage Jack to self-present to the student support services available through his university as you know they can offer counselling and support.

Huw Corness

Patient voice

'When my alarm goes off in the morning, I start to cry because I know my day is going to be filled with horrible thoughts, panic attacks and hours and hours of rituals. I cannot just turn off these feelings or rituals.'

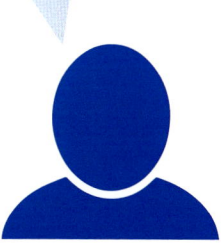

Do not do …

- Try not to reason with your patient about their illogical thinking and behaviour.
- Don't get involved with your patient's obsessions or rituals, this will make them worse.
- Don't bring up the topic of OCD repeatedly.
- It is not helpful to use the expression 'just try and relax …'

Recognising OCD

Obsessive-compulsive disorder (OCD) is an anxiety disorder (see Chapter 5 on Anxiety Disorders, p. 67), that is characterised by patients having distressing, repetitive thoughts. It can affect anyone regardless of age, gender, socioeconomic status or ethnicity (Mental Health Foundation, 2020). Once considered a neglected illness (Fineberg et al., 2020), OCD is now recognised as a common, highly disabling yet potentially treatable early-onset brain disorder. It is estimated that OCD occurs in about 1.1% of the general population in the UK according to the International OCD Foundation (2021). OCD has two main parts: obsessions and compulsions. Obsessions are described as unwelcome thoughts, urges, images, worries or doubts that repeatedly appear in the patient's mind. These obsessions can make patients feel anxious, although Mind (2020) describes it more as 'mental discomfort' than anxiety. The National Collaborating Centre for Mental Health (UK) (2006) gives the following examples and types of obsessions:

- A fear of causing or failure to prevent harm
- Intrusive thoughts
- Impulses and images
- Religious, or blasphemous, thoughts which are in conflict with the person's religion
- Fear of contamination
- Fears and worries related to order or symmetry.

Compulsions are repetitive actions that patients perform to reduce the feelings of discomfort or anxiety caused by the obsession (National Collaborating Centre for Mental Health (UK), 2006), for example, enacting rituals, checking, correcting thoughts and seeking reassurance.

On some days these obsessive compulsions are manageable but at other times patients will explain that they negatively affect their day-to-day lives. This is often influenced by the levels of stress patients feel around life changes, health, finances, work and relationships (Mind, 2020; National Institute of Mental Health, 2021). There is also an additional element – avoidance – which needs to be considered. Some activities or experiences can make OCD worse. Therefore, patients sometimes find it easier to avoid these situations. Unfortunately, as Heyman, Mataix-Cols and Fineberg (2006) also add, the shame and secrecy associated with OCD, as well as the lack of recognition of its symptoms, can lead to a delay in diagnosis and treatment.

Understanding OCD

As with many conditions, there are various causes and factors that contribute to OCD. According to the Mental Health Foundation (2020), exact causes are not fully understood. There are three likely factors that contribute to OCD: personal experiences, personality and biological factors (Mind, 2020). Interestingly, a study by Mataix-Cols et al. (2013) found that OCD clusters in families are primarily due to genetic factors.

The Mental Health Foundation (2020) adds that differences in the brain such as lower levels of serotonin or increased brain activity can contribute to OCD. Personal experiences, such as a painful childhood where trauma, abuse or bullying occurred, can cause some patients to start using obsessions or compulsions to cope with the anxiety triggered by past events. Further research into developmental factors and trauma-specific OCD is needed. Interestingly, there does seem to be a link between parents who have similar anxieties, thus showing similar kinds of compulsive behaviour which suggests that patients might have learned OCD behaviours as a coping mechanism (Mind, 2020). Ongoing stress and anxiety or being part of a stressful event such as a road traffic collision or starting a new job can trigger OCD or make it worse. Mind (2020) also suggests that pregnancy and giving birth can trigger perinatal OCD.

Personality is another possible contributing factor to OCD. Research suggests that people with certain personality traits may be more likely to have OCD; for example, if a person is meticulous, neat and methodical, with high standards, they are more likely to develop OCD (Huh et al., 2012). Biological factors such as the level of serotonin in the brain may also have an impact (Sinopoli, 2017). However, more research is needed to examine whether serotonin contributes to the cause or whether it is an effect of OCD (National Institute of Mental Health, 2021; Mind, 2020). Although genetics have also been considered, thus far, there are no conclusive outcomes from the research.

When considering diagnosis of OCD, be aware that people with OCD are often embarrassed by their condition and may not readily disclose all their symptoms. This might necessitate that you consider some direct questions about their symptoms. Patients may present with dermatological symptoms (from excessive washing), genital or anal symptoms (from excessive checking and washing) and stress (for example, from losing a job due to obsessive or compulsive behaviours). Consider screening patients with anxiety, alcohol or substance abuse, depression, or eating disorders as well as those who have symptoms which could suggest OCD. Possible questions might include the following: is the patient washing and cleaning a lot? Are they constantly checking things? Do they have any thoughts that keep bothering them that they wish they could get rid of? Do their daily activities take a long time to finish? Are they concerned about putting things in a certain order? Do they get upset by mess and, lastly, do these problems worry or trouble them? (NICE, 2018)

There are a multitude of other differential diagnoses to be aware of. According to NICE (2018) these include:

- Obsessive-compulsive personality disorder
- Body dysmorphic disorder
- Somatic symptom disorder
- Illness anxiety disorder (hypochondriasis)
- Delusional disorder
- Autism spectrum disorder (including Asperger's syndrome)
- Hoarding disorder
- Trichotillomania (hair-pulling disorder)
- Excoriation (skin-picking) disorder
- Substance-induced or medication-induced obsessive-compulsive disorder.

In addition, there are two types of diagnostic criterion for the diagnosis of OCD, the International Classification of Disease (ICD-11) and/or the *Diagnostic and Statistical Manual of Mental Disorders (DSM-5)*. Although paramedics are not expected to diagnose mental health conditions, it is helpful to understand how these conditions are diagnosed. The common diagnostic criteria across both classification systems includes that the patient has recurrent obsessional thoughts (persistent urges or impulses which are distressing, that are not part of another medical condition) and compulsive acts or rituals (repeated behaviour performed to prevent or reduce distress) (NICE, 2018).

Self-help ideas for your patient

Remember that OCD is distressing for your patient, and they may also be struggling to communicate and engage with others. It is therefore noteworthy that you can start your care of this patient with some supportive ideas to encourage their engagement in their condition. There are some physical activities you can suggest as well as some supportive tools which may help your patient reach out to others. A review into the effectiveness of self-help treatment by Mataix-Cols and Marks (2006) adds that self-help approaches have the potential to help many more patients who would otherwise remain inadequately treated or indeed, untreated.

Importance of physical wellbeing

Physical activity is vital in maintaining physical health. Consider advising your patient to do gentle activities such as yoga, swimming or walking as a starting point. Any kind of physical activity counts for something. Regular physical activity exerts positive effects on anxiety disorder symptoms, although the biological mechanisms underpinning this effect are not completely understood (Moylan et al., 2013).

Sleep is another important factor when considering your patient's physical health needs. Mind (2020) discusses the importance of adequate sleep as this can help patients cope with difficult feelings and experiences. Diet is often forgotten as another important element to physical health. Eating regularly ensures blood sugar levels remain stable as this can influence patients' mood and energy levels (Mind, 2020).

Reaching out to others

Finding other people with whom to discuss OCD is challenging because OCD is often difficult to talk about; patients will feel as though others may not understand what they are going through. The National Institute of Mental Health (2021) suggests encouraging patients to strengthen the relationships they already have as this will help with feeling lonely and unable to cope. Try to get patients to talk to someone they trust; some patients may also find it helpful to write down their feelings and then discuss them. Some patients may not be ready to share their thoughts and feelings, but spending time with family and friends may help them feel less isolated and more comfortable. In time, this may encourage them to share their feelings (Mind, 2020).

Self-help resources are designed to help patients develop coping strategies. Many resources are based on cognitive behavioural therapy (CBT) which is considered an effective treatment for OCD (Foa, 2010). Websites such as OCD-UK offer a range of helpful resources. You can also refer patients to their GP who can recommend appropriate reading material for OCD patients. There is a scheme called 'Books on Prescription' which is supported by most local libraries and also free to access. For more information about this scheme, visit https://reading-well.org.uk/books/books-on-prescription/mental-health/self-help (Reading Well, 2021). It's also important to point out that how patients perceive their condition can lead to important insights that would lead to improving their treatment (Pedley et al., 2019).

There is a variety of peer support available. Making connections and sharing experiences with people who feel the same is helpful. For the Mind infoline, or local Mind support group based on your geographical area, visit the Mind website for more information. There are also online peer support groups such as Elefriends, OCD-UK, OCD Actions and Top UK.

Reflective practices for your patient

There are a variety of ways that you can encourage patients to 'let go'. Managing stress levels is one way. Stress and anxiety make OCD worse and there are numerous ways of addressing this (Mind, 2020). Relaxation techniques are also useful and learning these can help patients to focus on their wellbeing whenever they are stressed, anxious and busy. Mindfulness has become more popular in recent years. Foa (2010) suggests that often CBT will include mindfulness as part of its therapeutic process. However, a study by Cludius et al. (2015) found that the effectiveness of mindfulness training as a self-help intervention was not supported, but they did add that there might be benefit in mindfulness for patients if delivered as therapist-guided intervention.

Clinical treatment and management

NICE (2018) has clear guidelines in terms of managing and monitoring patients with OCD. Which aspects are relevant to you depends on your clinical role and area of expertise. These guidelines are relevant for patients from eight years onwards. If your patient has received a diagnosis of OCD, assess the degree of their distress and functional impairment. NICE (2018) divides functional impairment into three categories: mild, moderate or severe. In order to assess this, ask the following questions: how are your symptoms affecting your work or school, relationships, your social life and quality of life. NICE (2018) also advises using the Yale-Brown Obsessive-Compulsive Scale (Y-BOCS), or questions derived from it to assess the severity of your patient's OCD. Again, you are not expected to diagnose OCD but it's important to understand how it is diagnosed and managed accordingly. This information may be useful when referring and discussing treatment plans with your patient.

Yale-Brown Obsessive-Compulsive Scale

This list of questions, from the Yale-Brown Obsessive-Compulsive Scale (Y-BOCS), is included as a guide. See Y-BOCS for a full symptom checklist according to NICE (2018), and visit med.stanford.edu/ocd/about/diagnosis.html for interpretation of the score.

The checklist includes the following questions:

- How much of your day is occupied by obsessive thoughts or spent performing compulsive acts (mild: less than one hour; moderate: one to three hours; severe: more than three hours)?

- How much do your obsessive thoughts or compulsive behaviours interfere with your social or work/school functioning (including relationships)?

- How much distress do your obsessive thoughts cause you? How would you feel if prevented from performing your compulsion(s)? How anxious would you become?

- How much of an effort do you make to resist the obsessive thoughts or compulsions?

- How much control do you have over your obsessive thoughts? How strong is the drive to perform the compulsions?

The Children's Y-BOCS (CY-BOCS) is similar to the adult version and can be used to assess the nature and severity of symptoms (NICE, 2018).

NICE (2018) suggests that OCD may exist alongside other mental health disorders such as depression, anxiety, alcohol or substance misuse, body dysmorphic disorder, and/or an eating disorder. It is imperative that if the patient is showing severe distress and/or functional impairment or other mental health co-morbidities, you also consider their risk of suicide and self-harm (NICE, 2018). For further information on the risk of suicide, see pp. 51–52 in Chapter 3 – Depression and the IPAP tool in Chapter 2 – Decision Making (p. 36).

> **Remember!**
>
> Don't forget to consider safeguarding concerns and complete the necessary referral forms relevant to your workplace to action this.

If uncertain, always seek the advice of mental health professionals with specific expertise in the assessment and management of OCD. NICE (2018) recommends discussing referral to specialist treatment for patients whose OCD is assessed as severe or where patients exhibit signs of being at risk of self-harm, self-neglect, a co-morbidity (such as substance misuse), severe depression, anorexia nervosa, or schizophrenia. Urgent (same day) referral to the crisis resolution and home treatment team is advised if the patient is at high risk of suicide.

If you are working in primary care, NICE (2018) suggests providing written material about OCD and its treatment options to your patient. These can be printed from a variety of appropriate resources such as Mind and the Royal College of Psychiatrists.

NICE (2018) recommends a psychological intervention for adults with mild functional impairment. This can be accessed by referral or self-referral to IAPT (Improving Access to Psychological Therapies). However, a recent study by Fisher et al. (2020) has shown that improvement in the efficacy of psychological interventions for patients is needed, as almost 80% of treated patients remain symptomatic.

For adults with moderate functional impairment (if you are confident of your assessment of moderate functional impairment), discuss the choice of intensive CBT or a selective serotonin reuptake inhibitor (SSRI). This will depend on your ability to assess moderate functional impairment, your area of clinical practice and your prescribing qualifications. If in doubt, NICE (2018) recommends referring your patient to the secondary care mental health team.

For adults with severe functional impairment, NICE (2018) advocates referring to the secondary care mental health team for assessment. Further details on additional considerations while waiting for assessment in secondary care can be found in the guidelines on the NICE website.

How should you monitor a patient with obsessive-compulsive disorder?

NICE (2018) reiterates the importance of being alert to suicidal ideation and ensuring you assess suicide risk, especially if your patient has co-morbid depression.

> **Remember!**
>
> Do not forget to consider factors such as severity and duration of symptoms, as well as the degree of distress and functional impairment.

Consider making use of the Y-BOCS scale, or questions originated from it, to compare with previous scores. Also check your patient's compliance to any treatment and ask about adverse drug effects (if applicable).

For patients in the initial stages of SSRI treatment, remember to ask about signs of akathisia or restlessness, suicidal ideation and increased anxiety and agitation. If they report prolonged akathisia, restlessness or agitation, consider a switch to a different SSRI and consult a senior clinician for further input if you are unsure how to proceed. Also advise your patient to report any cardiac symptoms such as palpitations, vertigo, syncope, or seizures if they are on clomipramine (NICE, 2018).

A study by Bloch et al. (2010) revealed that higher doses of SSRI are more effective in the treatment of adults with OCD. Higher doses of SSRIs than those suggested by NICE may be of additional benefit to some patients; this is something to discuss with the GP or area specialist.

References

Bloch M.H. et al. (2010). Meta-analysis of the dose-response relationship of SSRI in obsessive-compulsive disorder. *Molecular Psychiatry*, 15(8): 850–855.

Cludius B. et al. (2015). Mindfulness for OCD? No evidence for a direct effect of a self-help treatment approach. *Journal of Obsessive-Compulsive and Related Disorders*, 6: 59–65.

Fineberg N.A. et al. (2020). Clinical advances in obsessive-compulsive disorder: a position statement by the International College of Obsessive-Compulsive Spectrum Disorders. *International Clinical Psychopharmacology*, 35(4): 173–193.

Fisher P.L. et al. (2020). People with obsessive-compulsive disorder often remain symptomatic following psychological treatment: A clinical significance analysis of manualised psychological interventions. *Journal of Affective Disorders*, 275: 94–108.

Foa E.B. (2010). Cognitive behavioral therapy of obsessive-compulsive disorder. *Dialogues in Clinical Neuroscience*, 12(2): 199–207.

Heyman I., Mataix-Cols D. and Fineberg N.A. (2006). Obsessive-compulsive disorder, *British Medical Journal*, 333(7565): 424–429.

Huh M.J. et al. (2013). The Impact of Personality Traits on Ratings of Obsessive-Compulsive Symptoms. *Psychiatry Investigation*, 10(3): 259–265.

International OCD Foundation (2021). What is OCD? Available at: https://iocdf.org/about-ocd/

Mataix-Cols D. and Marks I.M. (2006). Self-help with minimal therapist contact for obsessive-compulsive disorder: a review, *European Psychiatry*, 21(2): 75–80.

Mataix-Cols D. et al. (2013). Population-Based, Multigenerational Family Clustering Study of Obsessive-compulsive Disorder. *JAMA Psychiatry*, 70(7): 709–717.

Mental Health foundation (2020). Obsessive-compulsive disorder (OCD). Available at: https://www.mentalhealth.org.uk/a-to-z/o/obsessive-compulsive-disorder-ocd

Mind (2020). Obsessive-compulsive disorder (OCD). Available at: https://www.Mind.org.uk/information-support/types-of-mental-health-problems/obsessive-compulsive-disorder-ocd/about-ocd/

Moylan S. et al. (2013). Exercising the worry away: How inflammation, oxidative and nitrogen stress mediates the beneficial effect of physical activity on anxiety disorder symptoms and behaviours, *Neuroscience & Biobehavioral Reviews*, 37(4): 573–584.

National Collaborating Centre for Mental Health (UK) (2006). *Obsessive-Compulsive Disorder: Core Interventions in the Treatment of Obsessive-Compulsive Disorder and Body Dysmorphic Disorder.* NICE Clinical Guidelines No. 31. Leicester: British Psychological Society.

National Institute of Mental Health (2021). Obsessive-Compulsive Disorder: When Unwanted Thoughts or Repetitive Behaviours Take Over. Available at: https://www.nimh.nih.gov/health/publications/obsessive-compulsive-disorder-when-unwanted-thoughts-take-over/

NICE (2018). Clinical Knowledge Summaries. Obsessive-compulsive disorder. Available at: https://cks.nice.org.uk/topics/obsessive-compulsive-disorder/

Pedley R., Bee P., Wearden A. and Berry K. (2019). Illness perceptions in people with obsessive-compulsive disorder: A qualitative study, *PLoS ONE*, 14(3): e0213495.

Reading Well (2021). Mental health. Available at: https://reading-well.org.uk/books/books-on-prescription/mental-health/self-help

Sinopoli V. (2017). A review of the role of serotonin system genes in obsessive-compulsive disorder. *Neuroscience & Biobehavioral Reviews*, 80: 372–381.

Post-Traumatic Stress Disorder

Ursula Rolfe

Case study

It's a cold, rainy Tuesday afternoon and you and your crew mate have just cleared from an incident. Without any downtime, you are dispatched to another call. Details are passed as '36-year-old male, unusual behaviour and seems anxious'.

On arrival, Lucy meets you at the door. She seems very upset and explains that she has called because she just doesn't know what to do for her husband Mark, who she thinks is having some kind of breakdown. Mark has recently left the army, having been a serving soldier for the last 10 years. His last tour was to Afghanistan where he witnessed one of his close friends, Tim, step on an IED. Tim survived but was severely injured.

You go upstairs to the first-floor flat and find Mark sitting on the sofa staring vacantly at the television. You approach cautiously and gently introduce yourself to him. Mark appreciates that you've taken time not to startle him, and in conversation, he shares with you that he has not been sleeping well for months and frequently has visual and audible memories of the incident which can occur at any time of the day or night, no matter what he is doing. He often feels startled by the memories because 'it feels like it's happening all over again'. Mark discloses that he thought his friend was going to die and was horrified by his injuries. He has questioned himself repeatedly, 'Why Tim? Why didn't it happen to me instead?' At this point, Mark becomes tearful.

Since the incident, Mark has been unable to concentrate or focus on everyday tasks. Lucy adds that her husband regularly seems as if he is 'miles away' but becomes distressed. At other times, Mark explained, 'stupid things' made him feel 'really angry, like I just can't contain it'.

Assessment

- Past medical history: normally fit and well. Has not seen his GP for years.
- Allergies: not disclosed.

- Drug history: none prescribed.
- Social history: lives with wife Lucy, no children. Unemployed after leaving the army six months ago. Using alcohol daily – limiting himself to 2 beers per day, smokes 10 cigarettes per day. Was running excessively but more recently has stopped going out.

On examination

- Appearance: Mark is dressed appropriately although he is unshaven. He looks exhausted and anxious. Appears to be of normal body weight.
- Behaviour: currently calm, engaging in the consultation with you. You are able to develop a rapport with him. Some appropriate eye contact but sometimes looks away/ into the distance.
- Speech/rapport with others: spontaneous conversation, able to understand what you are saying.
- Mood: despondent, hopeless, and confused as to what is happening to him. Easily tearful. Blames himself for Tim's injuries. Little interest in daily life – finds it difficult to concentrate and focus on tasks. Irritable, with moments of anger.
- Thoughts: thoughts are at a steady pace, are relevant to the circumstances and in a logical order. No delusions, obsessions or compulsions are revealed. No suicidal thoughts.
- Perception: Mark explains that he no longer feels like his 'old' self (pre-incident). He feels somewhat detached from life at times. He is aware that he probably requires further psychological support. You do not perceive that he may be at risk of serious harm to himself or others.
- Affect: general air of sadness, somewhat anxious although the intensity of his emotions comes across as somewhat flat.
- Cognition: Mark is orientated to time, date and place. He is rational in his thinking but finds it difficult to retain and remember things in the short term. Able to follow instructions.
- Insight and judgement: is aware that he is experiencing heightened emotions. Is aware that he is psychologically unwell but is confused as to why he is not coping with the traumatic incident. Understands that he probably requires further help.
- Risk: denies any suicidal thoughts or intention to harm himself or others. However he does make reference to 'life feeling like a continuous challenge' and 'I don't know how much longer I can go on like this for'.

Clinical observations

- Heart rate: 82 beats/min
- Blood pressure: 132/84 mmHg
- Blood glucose: 5.3 mml/l
- Respiratory rate: 14 breaths/min
- Temperature: Not taken
- SpO$_2$: 99% on room air

Questions for consideration

- What differential diagnoses are you considering?
- What are some of the challenges in handling this situation and how would you overcome them?
- What advice would you give to the patient? How would you manage the situation?

Impression

You believe that Mark may be experiencing post-traumatic stress disorder.

Plan

There are no red flags indicating any immediate risks to life. However, it is clear that Mark requires additional specialist psychological help. As it is a Tuesday afternoon, you gain Mark's consent to contact his own GP. You talk through Mark's history and presentation with the doctor who arranges to see Mark at the surgery that afternoon. The doctor explains that he will also make a referral to the community psychiatric team and put him in touch with a veterans' support charity.

Jo Mildenhall

Patient voice

'When I was diagnosed, I remember thinking that only military vets had that. But my doctor said that it could be triggered by any traumatising experience and that just one of these experiences separately could cause PTSD.'

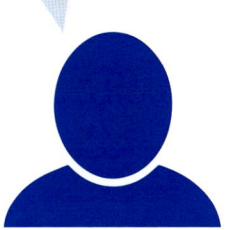

Do not do …

- Don't push for too much information too soon; this call will take time.

- Don't speak too loudly, as noise is often a trigger for those with PTSD.

- Don't question your patient's response to trauma: some may fight, others may experience flight, still others may freeze.

- Don't state or imply that your patient could have done something differently.

Recognising PTSD

Post-traumatic stress disorder (PTSD) is an anxiety disorder triggered by traumatic, frightening or distressing events as well as cumulative trauma exposure (NHS, 2020). One in two people experience trauma at some point in their lives with around 20% going on to develop PTSD (PTSDUK, 2020).

Patients with this disorder often relive these events through flashbacks and nightmares and can also experience feeling isolated, irritable and guilty. According to Grinage (2003), PTSD used to be called 'shell shock' during World War I, 'war neurosis' in World War II and 'combat stress reaction' during the Vietnam War. PTSDUK (2020) adds that the majority of patients who are exposed to traumatic events experience some short-term distress which can resolve without professional intervention; however a small proportion who develop the disorder are unlikely to seek out help. Interestingly, 70% of patients who have PTSD in the UK do not receive any professional therapeutic input and their quality of life is substantially reduced (PTSDUK, 2020). Exposure to a traumatic event can occur in one or more ways: the patient experiences the traumatic event; they witness, in person, the traumatic event; and they learn that someone close to them experienced, or was part of, a traumatic event. Interestingly, epidemiologic studies from around the world have demonstrated that most people in the community have experienced traumatic events that would fulfil stressor criterion for PTSD (Sareen, 2014).

According to Mind (2020), PTSD may be described differently in some situations. For example, delayed-onset PTSD could be applicable if your patient's symptoms emerge more than six months after experiencing a trauma; this might be described as 'delayed PTSD' or 'delayed-onset PTSD'. There is also the condition called complex PTSD. This occurs if your patient experienced trauma at an early age or it lasted for a long time. The final type of PTSD is called 'birth trauma': PTSD which develops after a traumatic experience of childbirth.

It is important to consider who is more at risk of PTSD. There are several factors to take into account when considering this, including (Mind, 2020):

- Whether your patient is experiencing repeated trauma

- Whether they are in pain or getting physically hurt

- Whether your patient has little or no support from friends, family or professionals

- Whether your patient is experiencing additional stress at the same time

- Whether your patient has previously experienced anxiety or depression.

Results from the WHO World Mental Health (WMH) surveys published by Kessler et al. (2017) reveal that PTSD due to trauma exposure has a longer mean symptom duration than was previously thought and this means that it is vital to take risk factors into account when recognising PTSD.

When recognising PTSD, it's also important to consider the concept of post-traumatic growth (PTG). PTG is defined as a positive psychological change experienced due to coping with challenging life circumstances or trauma and it is often associated with mental health recovery (Slade et al., 2019).

Understanding PTSD

Although it is not your role to diagnose PTSD, understanding the criteria for diagnosis is helpful in understanding the condition. The *DSM-5* outlines three domains of symptoms to consider pertaining to a diagnosis of PTSD: re-experiencing, avoidance and hyperarousal (American Psychiatric Association, 2013). These symptoms include your patient:

- Re-experiencing a traumatic event through 'flashbacks' or having dreams/ nightmares

- Feeling defeated or worthless

- Having problems in relationships

- Experiencing emotional dysregulation

- Feeling disconnected

- Lacking the ability to experience feelings and feeling detached from other people

- Giving up activities that they have previously enjoyed

- Communicating less with others

- Negative alterations in mood and thinking

- Hyperarousal

- Avoiding situations that trigger memories of the traumatic event.

PTSD should be considered in people presenting with depression, anxiety disorders and problems with substance abuse. NICE (2020) recommends considering the differential diagnoses of PTSD and awareness that PTSD may be co-morbid with some of these conditions, particularly depression and anxiety disorders. PTSD should also be considered in patients repeatedly presenting with unexplained physical symptoms. A review by Pacella, Hruska and Delahanty (2013) showed that there was a relationship between PTSD and general physical symptoms. Physical symptoms such as headaches, gastrointestinal issues, rheumatic pains and skin disorders should be considered when considering a diagnosis of PTSD. You should also be aware of occupations and lifestyle factors that may be risk factors for exposure to traumatic events and the development of PTSD. According Skogstad et al. (2013) professionals such as police officers, firefighters and ambulance personnel often experience incidents that satisfy the stressor criterion for the PTSD diagnosis. Other professional groups such as health care professionals, train drivers, divers, journalists, sailors and employees in banks, post offices or in stores may also be subjected to work-related traumatic events. Work-related PTSD usually diminishes with time.

Clinicians may find the use of a validated screening questionnaire useful when considering a diagnosis of PTSD. Using a tool may also be beneficial for patients deemed at high risk of PTSD (NICE, 2020). As paramedics are not required to diagnose mental health conditions, always consider discussing your patient and their symptoms with a suitably qualified colleague. In most cases, referral to a mental health specialist with expertise in managing post-traumatic stress disorder is required. According to NICE (2020), they usually make a diagnosis using diagnostic criteria from the fifth edition of the American Psychiatric Association's *Diagnostic and Statistical Manual of Mental Disorders (DSM-5)* or the International Classification of Diseases (ICD-11); this will be discussed a little later in more detail.

If you are working in primary care, NICE (2020) suggests using the Trauma Screening Questionnaire (TSQ) which consists of 10 questions which measure re-experiencing and arousal symptoms. Remember, it is designed to be used three weeks or more following exposure to a traumatic event to identify patients who are likely to be currently suffering from post-traumatic stress disorder. It will ask which symptoms your patient has experienced at least twice in the past week. A recent study by De Bont et al. (2018) into the validity of the TSQ for PTSD among patients with psychotic disorders showed it to be valid and useful. This free questionnaire may be accessed via the NICE website.

As well as considering a diagnosis, as usual in clinical practice, it is advisable to also consider differential diagnoses in terms of patients presenting with possible PTSD. NICE (2020) suggests considering the following conditions as alternative differential diagnoses: depression, generalised anxiety disorder, phobias, dissociative disorders and psychosis.

For a patient to be diagnosed by an appropriate clinician, they must meet specific diagnostic criteria according to two sources, either using the fifth edition of the American Psychiatric Association's *Diagnostic and Statistical Manual of Mental Disorders (DSM-5)* or the International Classification of Diseases (ICD-11). For further information on these sources and their criteria, visit the NICE (2020) PTSD guidelines.

Self-help ideas for your patient

Remember that PTSD is a difficult experience for your patient, and they may also be struggling to communicate and engage with others. It is therefore noteworthy that you can start your care of this patient with some supportive ideas to encourage their engagement in their condition. In fact, a recent study by Lewis et al. (2017) found that internet-based, trauma-focused, guided self-help for PTSD was a favourable treatment option. There are some helpful tips you can suggest as well as some supportive tools which may help your patient.

Physical health

Remember that coping with PTSD can be exhausting. Patients will sometimes experience low energy levels which is why you need to ensure they are also taking the following elements into consideration: a healthy diet with regular meals to ensure stable blood sugar; physical activity to help improve mood and energy levels which can include spending time outdoors. They should also avoid drugs or alcohol (Mind, 2020). In fact, a study by Walton et al. (2018) looked at the relationship between *DSM-5* PTSD symptom clusters and alcohol misuse among military veterans; they found that there was a positive association between alcohol abuse and PTSD symptom severity. Increased alcohol consumption may therefore interfere with treatments for PTSD.

Many patients who experience PTSD have difficulties with sleeping. They may find it hard to fall or stay asleep, feel unsafe during the night, or anxious and afraid of having nightmares. Advise them on proper sleep hygiene and consider referring them to their GP for a hypnotic medication for short-term use (NICE, 2020). Whitworth et al. (2019) add that high-intensity resistance training (HIRT) improves sleep quality and anxiety in adults with PTSD.

Tips on coping with flashbacks

Patients can find that certain experiences, situations or people seem to trigger flashbacks or other symptoms. These might include specific reminders of past trauma, such as smells, sounds, words, places or particular types of books or films. Some patients find things especially difficult on significant dates, such as the anniversary of a traumatic experience (Mind, 2020).

Flashbacks can be very distressing, but there are things you can suggest to your patient that might help. Feelings of panic and fear lead to abnormal breathing patterns so focusing on breathing helps to regulate those patterns. They could also carry something that will remind them of the present instead of the past. Your patient could also comfort themselves by listening to soothing music, cuddling their pet, or snuggling up in a blanket.

Reaching out to others

People who experience PTSD may find it hard to open up to others. This may be because they feel unable to talk about what happened to them. Remind them that they don't need to describe a trauma to tell someone how they are currently feeling. Encourage them to talk to a friend, or their family, or refer them to their GP for further talking therapy advice and referrals (Mind, 2020). Peer support brings together people who have had similar experiences, which some people find very helpful; peer support groups can be found by visiting the Mind website.

Reflective practices for your patient

Everyone has their own unique response to trauma, and it is important for patients to take things at their own pace. For example, it may not be helpful to talk about their experiences before they feel ready. Remind them to be patient with themselves and not to judge themselves harshly for needing time and support to recover from PTSD. They could also start a diary and make notes of what happens when they experience a flashback so that they can understand their patterns and potential triggers. This will help them to identify signs as they begin to emerge.

Specialist support

There is a large network online for different specialist support mechanisms. Encourage patients to look into these websites so that they can find support to suit their individual needs. There is also specialist support information on the UK Psychological Trauma Society website.

Clinical treatment and management

NICE has clear guidelines in terms of managing and monitoring patients with PTSD. In primary care, the lead role will be that of the GP. However, it is always good to understand the guidelines that the GP will be following when making treatment decisions in support of the patient. According to NICE (2020), the main role of the GP in the initial management of a patient with symptoms of PTSD will be to determine whether there is a need for an emergency physical and mental health assessment and then to coordinate appropriate care. It is likely that when a referral to specialist treatment such as psychological therapy or drug treatment is made, there will be a waiting period. Also, remember where confirmation of the diagnosis has taken place in primary care and whether specialist referral is required for any further management (NICE, 2020). NICE (2020) recommends the GP assess the patient as follows:

For all patients with symptoms of PTSD, NICE suggests asking about its effects on work or school, relationships, social life and quality of life, in order to assess the degree of distress and functional impairment as mild, moderate, or severe. Mild is defined as 'distress caused by the symptoms is manageable, and the person's social and occupational functioning are not significantly impaired'. Moderate is described as 'distress and impact on functioning [lying] somewhere between mild and severe [...] there is not considered to be a significant risk of suicide, harm to self, or harm to others' and last, severe distress 'caused by the symptoms is felt to be unmanageable, and/or there is significant impairment in social and/or occupational functioning, and/or there is considered to be significant risk of suicide, harm to self, or harm to others'.

NICE (2020) highlights the fact that clinically important symptoms of PTSD can be defined as those causing at least moderate functional impairment and/or those scoring above a clinical threshold on a validated scale which has been used to assess a patient. Where symptoms are considered moderate, NICE (2020) advises GPs to use their clinical judgement to determine the need for intervention.

In addition, NICE (2020) guides clinicians to also be aware that PTSD can commonly co-exist with other mental health disorders such as depression, anxiety disorders and alcohol or substance misuse. If the patient is showing severe signs of distress or functional impairment or has co-morbidities such as depression or another health disorder, it is recommended that the patient be assessed for suicide risk and self-harm. See pp. 51–52 in Chapter 3 – Depression and the IPAP tool in Chapter 2 – Decision Making (p. 36). If your patient is considered high risk, they should be referred urgently and on the same day to the crisis resolution and home treatment team.

> **Remember!**
>
> Do not forget to consider any safeguarding issues.

If the patient does not require a same-day referral, consider the following additional elements. If your patient has co-morbid depression, be aware that treating PTSD first is often associated with an improvement in depression. But, if your patient's depression is severe enough to make psychological treatment of the PTSD difficult, the depression should be treated first. Also carry out a physical health assessment if your patient has any physical health concerns or there are red flags.

> **Remember!**
>
> Do not forget to assess your patient's social needs and then make appropriate referrals accordingly (NICE, 2020).

NICE (2020) recommends that for patients with clinically notable PTSD symptoms where a traumatic event has occurred within the last month, clinicians should initiate specialist referral for psychological therapy or drug treatment. For those with clinically important PTSD symptoms that have continued for more than one month after a traumatic event, offer referral to a specialist mental health service for psychological therapy or drug treatment. Be aware that availability and arrangements for accessing trauma-focused psychological treatments may vary locally, and there may sometimes be a significant delay before treatment begins.

If an (adult) patient prefers drug treatment, declines referral for psychological therapies or referral is significantly delayed, NICE (2020) suggests prescribing antidepressants such as venlafaxine or an SSRI. Salas et al. (2020) suggest that PSTD is associated with poor antidepressant medication adherence. Their study also adds that earlier literature suggests antidepressant medication adherence improves depression symptoms; therefore PTSD symptom reduction may lead to better depression outcomes. Visit the NICE website for further details on adverse effects, withdrawal symptoms and review processes.

Psychological therapies and drug treatment

Specialists may offer a patient with PTSD trauma-focused psychological treatments which are considered first-line (NICE, 2020). Another alternative is trauma-focused cognitive behavioural therapy (CBT) which consists of a combination of exposure therapy and trauma-focused cognitive therapy. However, more complicated presentations will probably require longer treatment. Internet-based CBT offers alternative and more accessible treatment for those with PTSD. According to Simon et al. (2019) this appears to be an acceptable intervention for adults with PTSD.

Exposure therapy can also be effective (NICE, 2020). Exposure therapy is where your patient confronts traumatic memories (usually by recounting the event) and is also repeatedly exposed to situations which they have been avoiding in order to elicit fear. Prolonged exposure therapy can be an effective treatment for PTSD if the therapist ensures that fear is appropriately activated and negative cognitions are identified and modified (Brown, Zandberg and Foa, 2019).

Trauma-focused cognitive therapy identifies and modifies misrepresentations of the trauma and its aftermath that lead the patient to overestimate threat (NICE, 2020).

NICE (2020) also recommends eye movement desensitisation and reprocessing (EMDR) and advises up to 12 sessions with more complex presentations likely to require longer treatment. EMDR uses bilateral stimulation – eye movements, taps, and tones – while the patient focuses on memories and associations in order to help the brain process flashbacks and to make sense of the traumatic experience. Bae et al. (2018) add that EMDR can be a successful add-on after failure of initial pharmacotherapy for PTSD.

Recommendations for treating sleep disturbance are pragmatic based on what NICE (2020) considers to be good clinical practice and in keeping with NICE's recommendation that the initial assessment of a patient with PTSD should be comprehensive, including an assessment of physical and psychological needs.

Recommendations for follow-up and monitoring of the patient's symptoms, functioning and response to treatment at intervals should be pragmatic and determined by clinical judgement and as part of any shared care arrangement (if applicable).

References

American Psychiatric Association (2013). Diagnostic and Statistical Manual of Mental Disorders (DSM-5), *Fifth Edition*. Washington, DC: American Psychiatric Association Publishing, 87–120.

Bae H. et al. (2018). Add-on Eye Movement Desensitization and Reprocessing (EMDR) Therapy for Adults with Post-traumatic Stress Disorder Who Failed to Respond to Initial Antidepressant Pharmacotherapy, *Journal of Korean Medical Science*, 33(48): e306.

Brown L.A., Zandberg L.J. and Foa E.B. (2019). Mechanisms of change in prolonged exposure therapy for PTSD: Implications for clinical practice. *Journal of Psychotherapy Integration*, 29(1): 6–14.

De Bont P. et al. (2015). Predictive validity of the Trauma Screening Questionnaire in detecting post-traumatic stress disorder in patients with psychotic disorders. *British Journal of Psychiatry*, 206(5): 408–416.

Grinage B.D. (2003). Diagnosis and management of post-traumatic stress disorder. *American Family Physician*, 68(12): 2401–2408.

Kessler R.C. et al. (2017). Trauma and PTSD in the WHO World Mental Health Surveys. *European Journal of Psychotraumatology*, 8(Sup.5): 1353383.

Lewis C.E. et al. (2017). Internet-based guided self-help for post-traumatic stress disorder (PTSD): randomised controlled trial. *Depression and Anxiety*, 34(6): 555–565.

Mind (2020). Post-traumatic stress disorder (PTSD). Available at: https://www.mind.org.uk/information-support/types-of-mental-health-problems/post-traumatic-stress-disorder-ptsd/self-care-for-ptsd/

NHS (2020). Overview – Post-traumatic stress disorder (PTSD). Available at: https://www.nhs.uk/conditions/post-traumatic-stress-disorder-ptsd/

NICE (2020). Clinical Knowledge Summaries. Post-traumatic stress disorder – Diagnosis – When should I suspect post-traumatic stress disorder (PTSD)? Available at: https://cks.nice.org.uk/post-traumatic-stress-disorder#!diagnosisSub

Pacella M.L., Hruska B. and Delahanty D.L. (2013). The physical health consequences of PTSD and PTSD symptoms: A meta-analytic review. *Journal of Anxiety Disorders*, 27(1): 33–46.

PTSDUK (2020). What is Post Traumatic Stress Disorder? Available at: https://www.ptsduk.org/what-is-ptsd/?gclid=EAIaIQobChMIm5uyk7ua6QIV5IBQBh37OQxZEAAYAiAAEgLga_D_BwE

Salas J. et al. (2020). Large posttraumatic stress disorder improvement and antidepressant medication adherence. *Journal of Affective Disorders*, 260: 119–123.

Sareen J. (2014). Posttraumatic Stress Disorder in Adults: Impact, Comorbidity, Risk Factors, and Treatment. *Canadian Journal of Psychiatry*, 59(9): 460–467.

Simon N. et al. (2019). Acceptability of internet-based cognitive behavioural therapy (i-CBT) for post-traumatic stress disorder (PTSD): a systematic review. *European Journal of Psychotraumatology*, 10(1): 1646092.

Skogstad M. et al. (2013). Work-related post-traumatic stress disorder. *Occupational Medicine*, 63(3): 175–182.

Slade M. et al. (2019). Post-traumatic growth in mental health recovery: qualitative study of narratives. *BMJ Open*, 9: e029342.

Walton, J.L., et al. (2018). The relationship between DSM-5 PTSD symptom clusters and alcohol misuse among military veterans. *American Journal on Addictions*, 27(1): 23–28.

Whitworth J.W., Nosrat S., SantaBarbara N.J. and Ciccolo J.T. (2019). High intensity resistance training improves sleep quality and anxiety in individuals who screen positive for posttraumatic stress disorder: A randomized controlled feasibility trial. *Mental Health and Physical Activity*, 16: 43–49.

Psychosis and Schizophrenia

Ursula Rolfe

Case study

It is a Friday night and the beginning of your shift. You are assigned the following case, which is typical for a front-line ambulance: 'Acute Psychosis', to transport from a local police custody centre to a secure mental health unit. The patient is male, 40 years old. You are dispatched as a Category 3 response – a two-hour average wait according to NHS England (2018). The transfer is requested by the Mental Health Crisis team who have placed him under Section 2 while in police custody.

On arrival, the custody sergeant gives a handover. The patient was brought to the attention of the police at approximately 06.00 hours. The police found him naked outside his flat having inflicted significant damage to the property and the surrounding area. Police took him into custody where he was detained for criminal damage. The mental health crisis team was contacted to assess. The subsequent Section 2 paperwork left for you, as the transporting ambulance crew, includes assessment and a brief past medical history. The crisis team did not attend until about 17:30 hours, referral for transport to a secure unit was ordered at approximately 20:30 hours.

The police tell you that the patient had not coped well in custody. He had torn up books, pushed his socks down the toilet, flooded the cell and washed himself repeatedly with water from the in-cell cistern. A custody officer arrives with the patient. From the Section 2 paperwork and your interactions with the patient, you obtain the following information:

Assessment

- Past medical history: the patient was known to mental health services but recorded as not engaging with community teams at present.
- Allergies: none.
- Drug history: the patient admits to non-compliance with medication.
- Social history: lives alone, unsupported accommodation, sister described as supportive by patient but not local.

On examination

- Appearance: despite your expectations from the history given by custody staff, he is brought to you and appears tidy and organised.

- Behaviour: friendly, compliant and calm, although skin is flushed. During physical assessment this flushing spreads to chest and neck, accompanied by sweating, tachycardia and reports of nausea. On the way to hospital he occasionally dry retches into a bowl. You notice that a fine tremor develops when you move on to blood glucose monitoring. The tension displayed resolves when physical examination is suspended. Interaction with him is in part to calm him in order to acquire the baseline observations needed to rule out any other medical concerns that should be assessed at the hospital in the emergency department (ED).

- Speech: clear, not slurred, excellent ability to communicate, he speaks freely, is engaging and articulate.

- Mood: jovial though tense, at times confused and distracted.

- Thoughts: en route, he tells you what it is like going to ED and being there with psychosis. They are fractured, indirect images of his experiences. He describes hallucinations, confusion over who is who, misunderstanding what is being communicated to him, noise, confusion from fragments of conversation overheard, mistrust regarding medication and unanswered questions. When performing baseline observations, the patient abruptly makes reference to having had similar tests before and he confesses that he is never told why, that he cannot think why thereby demonstrating suspicion.

- Perception: distorted, irrational beliefs about his body being unclean and subject to supposition. Admits to hallucinations visual, auditory and olfactory.

- Affect: patient was tending toward positive evaluation of present experience except when it came to physical contact and assessment which appeared to trigger a sympathetic response prompting the patient to admit feelings of doubt in your role.

- Cognition: scope narrowed at times of stress (during physical assessment) and broadened when relaxed.

- Insight and judgement: patient insight was fair, in that he recognised that he had mental ill health. Patient was compliant with the process through being sectioned, but did not seem entirely sure of his events being pathological. He accepted his judgement to make sound, reasonable and responsible decisions was impaired, but was capable of expressing distrust in decisions made for him.

- Risk: medium. The patient was of large build, clearly tense, with a history of physically destructive behaviour. However, police reported no physical violence toward staff and compliance while in custody. Looking back through his police record, they confirmed that there were no physical violence markers towards people.

- Scoring: using the Brief Psychiatric Rating Scale (Overall and Gorham, 1962), he scored highly. His 'somatic concern' was severe. In between pleasant, richly varied conversation, he interjects concerns about his body 'you see I have this umbilical hernia ...' and he shows his navel, with reddened skin, synonymous with self-infliction; 'I just don't know where it goes to, that's the thing' and he stares at it with fixed concern, then replaces his t-shirt and looks up, smiles and changes the subject.

Clinical observations

- Heart rate: 107 beats/min
- Blood pressure: 154/89 mmHg
- Blood glucose: 5.6. mmL/l
- Respiratory rate: 20 breaths/min
- Temperature: 36.8°C
- SpO_2: 99% on room air

The transport arrangements were without police escort. The ambulance arrives at the secure unit at about 22:00 hours; however the patient is not admitted into the building until approximately 23:00 hours, due to confusion at the secure unit regarding bed spaces. Another delay, a total of 17 hours from first contact with police. It took nearly 12 hours to be assessed by a mental health crisis team. NICE guidelines (2011) state that a patient in crisis should be assessed within four hours. It is a poor start to treatment but not unfamiliar, the negative effects of delays as well as the inappropriateness of police custody have been noted in research (Daggenvoorde, Gijsman and Goossens, 2018).

Questions for consideration

- What differentiates psychosis from a personality disorder when observing this patient's experiences?
- Consider baseline observations that would alert you to recommend emergency department assessment prior to arriving at the mental health facility. What alternative diagnosis might be possible?
- How could you better manage this patient's experience of hospitalisation?
- What would you change about the process if you could?

Impression

Psychosis

Plan

As a crew with a patient such as this, the best treatment is to listen as what you hear greatly enriches understanding. By explaining what you are doing, by constantly reaffirming the importance of his consent, you can work with what compliance the patient affords. Transparency was key in this case study.

Another important role of the crew member is as patient advocate at the secure unit, liaising with staff as they resolve any organisational issues, trying to smooth the already bumpy passage of the patient in his journey through crisis.

Discussion

In acute presentations of psychosis, it is rare to have a patient that communicates as generously and revealingly, reminiscent of an article published in the *British Medical Journal* (2015) by an anonymous author also suffering with episodes of acute psychosis. They tell of the difficulties in understanding doctors and clinicians when in crisis, of trust/mistrust, the challenge of coping with noise, the practical implications of sleep deprivation, good questioning styles, and good/bad posture or body language. They write 'In my experience, the best communicators use calm and clarity; they treat the distressed person as a person. Paramedics are often good at this.'

Sarah-Jane Niles

Patient voice

'I thought I was under constant surveillance and that everyone was out to get me. The radio, the TV, newspapers – they all spoke to me. But this doesn't mean I am going to kill you ...'

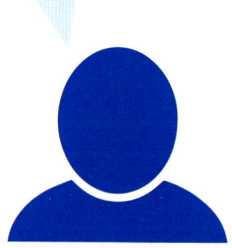

Do not do...

- If the patient is struggling to concentrate, keep your statements or questions short.

- Don't argue with the patient; accept their reality.

- Don't crowd or rush your patient; this will agitate them further.

- Don't reason with someone in acute psychosis; they cannot think rationally during this time.

Recognising psychosis and schizophrenia

We first need to consider the terms psychosis and schizophrenia separately. Psychosis is a syndrome embedded in several disorders, including schizophrenia and bipolar disorder with psychotic features (Lieberman and First, 2018). There seems to be much confusion about what it means to experience psychosis. There is often the assumption that if a patient is psychotic they are dangerous; this is not always the case and there remains a great deal of stigma associated with this symptom. Mental Health First Aid (2020) reveals that 6% of the population say they have experienced at least one symptom of psychosis. According to NICE (2020), psychosis and the diagnosis of schizophrenia characterise 'a major psychiatric disorder' where a patient's thoughts, mood, behaviour and perceptions are changed drastically. Thirty-eight per cent of people recover after a first episode of psychosis, and symptoms improve for 58% of people (Mental Health First Aid, 2020).

Schizophrenia is a mental disorder that causes psychosis, but it also has other symptoms and it isn't the only cause of psychosis. According to BMJ Best Practice (2021), it is characterised by a co-occurrence of at least two of the following symptoms: delusions, hallucinations, disorganised speech, disorganised/catatonic behaviour, or negative symptoms (e.g. affective flattening, avolition, anhedonia, attention deficit, or impoverishment of speech and language) occurring for a significant period of at least one month and associated with continuous problems over at least a six-month period. Interestingly, males have a higher risk of developing schizophrenia during their lifetime (Mental Health First Aid, 2020).

Other causes of psychosis include depression, bipolar disorder, dementia and borderline personality disorder. According to the American Psychiatric Association (2021) there are misconceptions around schizophrenia that are important to be aware of. The condition is often misunderstood and many people have negative views and assumptions about the condition. Mind (2020) reiterates that being diagnosed with schizophrenia does not mean the patient has a 'split personality'. Some people think hearing voices means that person is dangerous, but according to Mind (2020) when patients hear voices they are actually more likely to harm themselves than someone else.

Like so many mental health conditions, the cause of schizophrenia is not known; therefore treatment focuses on the symptoms. However, researchers believe there are contributing factors which according to NHS (2021) include a combination of physical, genetic, psychological and environmental factors. Links have been drawn between schizophrenia and substance abuse (Winklbaur et al., 2006). Apart from alcohol misuse, substances commonly abused include nicotine, cocaine and cannabis (Winklbaur et al., 2006). There has also been a link to the levels of dopamine in the brain, with patients diagnosed with schizophrenia having higher levels of this chemical. In most cases, schizophrenia is an end result of a complex interaction between thousands of genes and multiple environmental risk factors – none of which on their own causes schizophrenia (Gilmore, 2020).

Understanding psychosis and schizophrenia

Remember, it is not the role of the paramedic to diagnose these conditions, but if you have an understanding of the signs, symptoms and management, this will help you to signpost your patient to the appropriate healthcare professionals. The *DSM-5* (American Psychiatric Association, 2013) has clear diagnostic criteria which include the presence of two or more of the following (each present for a significant amount of time during a one-month period: delusions, hallucinations, disorganised speech, grossly disorganised or catatonic behaviour and negative symptoms. Interestingly, one study claims there is a possibility to classify schizophrenic patients and healthy controls using network properties and that there is a provisional pattern of the brain regions involved among patients with schizophrenia (Jo et al., 2020).

As well as considering how these patients are diagnosed, use your clinical judgement and also consider differential diagnoses. These include (NICE, 2020):

- Severe depression or bipolar disorder with psychotic symptoms
- Drug-induced psychosis often caused by opioids, cocaine, amphetamines and cannabis
- Sepsis
- Other primary medical conditions such as cerebral tumours, epilepsy or cerebrovascular disease
- PTSD
- OCD
- Communication or autism spectrum disorders.

Self-help ideas for your patient

Remember that experiencing psychosis and schizophrenia can be a traumatising experience for your patient, and they may also be struggling to communicate and engage with others. It is therefore noteworthy that you can start your care of this patient with some supportive ideas to encourage their engagement in their condition. Internet-based, CBT-orientated interventions provide an add-on effect to care as usual and have the potential to narrow the psychological treatment gap in psychosis (Westermann et al., 2020). There are other tips you can suggest as well as some supportive tools which may help your patient reach out to others.

Physical health

Getting enough sleep is very important when it comes to physical health. It helps make patients feel calmer and therefore, more able to cope. Try to encourage patients to eat a balanced diet as eating regularly helps avoid psychosis being brought on by changes in blood glucose levels (Mind, 2020). If a patient is on antipsychotic medication, they should be advised not to smoke as smoking can influence the effects of antipsychotic drugs. Alcohol and recreational drugs may also affect medication. Research shows that patients with schizophrenia and related psychoses often use, abuse and become dependent on psychoactive substances (Margolese et al., 2004).

Reflective practices for your patient

Mind (2020) advises that excessive stress can exacerbate symptoms of schizophrenia. An awareness of this is important, therefore, consider advising patients to seek out de-stressing activities. Also talk to your patient about what kind of responsibilities they have and whether they might be lessened by looking at support services in their area.

It might help patients to plan ahead for difficult times. Sit down with your patient and discuss how they would want to be helped again should they feel unwell.

Reaching out to others

It's important to do things that will help the patient boost their confidence levels. A focus on practical things helps to calm the mind. Feeling connected to other people is also an important factor in staying well. Feeling isolated and lonely can make symptoms worse (Mind, 2020). Suggest support services or peer support local to the patient for more advice; peer support can be useful as it brings together patients with similar experiences. Visit the Mind website or search the internet for peer support directories. There are also online forums such as Elefriends that can assist with your patient's needs.

Encourage patients to be aware of triggers or warning signs related to their condition. Although these triggers may be slightly different for everyone, some common signs that may cause your patient to spiral may include: feeling particularly anxious or stressed, sleeping badly, feeling scared or suspicious, hearing voices, difficulty in concentrating and becoming more isolated (Mind, 2020). Resilience is important in understanding thoughts and behaviours of patients with schizophrenia, especially if they are suicidal (Harris et al., 2020). Pay attention to these triggers and don't forget to encourage your patient to ask for help. Attendance at appointments is also important.

Clinical treatment and management

According to NICE (2020) part of managing psychosis and schizophrenia is the consideration of patients most at risk of developing a psychotic disorder or experiencing psychosis. NICE (2020) advises that a patient presenting with hallucinations and delusions, lack of spontaneity or reactive mood, lack of drive, lack of pleasure, attention deficit or changes in speech and language should be considered at risk of having psychosis. For further information about identifying risks, consult the NICE Clinical Guidelines (NICE, 2011) and refer your patient to their GP or mental health specialist for further clarification, assessment and management.

For all patients at risk of developing a psychotic disorder and those with psychotic symptoms, NICE (2020) advises undertaking an assessment of the risk of harm to the patient and/or others. Consideration of the following is recommended:

- Do they have a history of self-harm?
- Do they have suicidal ideation and plans?
- Do they feel hopeless?
- Do they misuse drugs and/or alcohol?
- Is there is a risk of accidental or non-accidental injury?
- If the patient is experiencing 'command' hallucinations, do they feel compelled to act upon them?
- What is their level of family/social support and how regularly are they in contact with support networks.

According to NICE (2020) the highest risk of suicide tends to be around the time of a psychotic episode and shortly after hospital discharge. (Also refer to the section on assessing the risk of suicide in Chapter 3 –Depression (pp. 51–52) and the IPAP tool in Chapter 2 – Decision Making (p. 36).

NICE (2020) also adds that clinicians should assess the patient's risk of unintentional harm to themselves caused by disorganised behaviour or poor judgement of risk due to their absorption with psychotic experiences and beliefs. To do this, NICE (2020) advises that you determine the patient's risk of harm to others by asking the patient about their social circumstance and carer responsibilities.

Remember!

Don't forget to follow your local safeguarding procedures where necessary.

Consider whether they are a risk to the public, especially if there is a previous history of public risk. Always consider your own safety – which must come first. Find out whether your patient is experiencing delusions focused on a particular individual.

> **Remember!**
>
> Don't forget to think about the risk from others including any adult safeguarding issues, for example, vulnerability to traumatic injuries, accidents, assault, or exploitation.

For those judged to be at high risk of harm to themselves or others, NICE (2020) recommends arranging a same-day specialist mental health assessment by the Early Intervention in Psychosis (EIP) service. If this service is not available and the risk of the patient or others is considered to exceed the management capacity of the EIP team, refer the patient to a crisis resolution and home treatment team. If they need to be admitted, try to persuade them to go voluntarily (NICE, 2020). However, if they decline, compulsory admission may be necessary under Sections 2 or 4 of the Mental Health Act (1983). Refer to mental health specialists such as social workers, community mental health nurses, GP and police for further advice.

If the patient is not thought to present a high risk of harm to themselves or others, refer them for specialist assessment. The patient should *not* be started on antipsychotic drug treatment while awaiting specialist assessment unless under advice from a consultant psychiatrist (NICE, 2020). A longitudinal study showed that antipsychotic medications do not remove or reduce the frequency of psychosis in schizophrenia (Harrow, Jobe and Faull, 2014). For your awareness, and if you work in primary care, the recommended support for ongoing primary care management includes monitoring the patient's symptoms, and if applicable, following crisis plans developed in secondary care and liaising with secondary care specialists (NICE, 2020). Review your patient's physical health, mental health and medication (if appropriate to your clinical role) at least annually, and more often if the patient, carer or healthcare professional has any concerns. Also ask your patient about their support structure and availability and consider referral to the community mental health service for family intervention to manage any conflict or difficulties that could trigger a relapse. Lastly, NICE (2020) adds that you need to ensure that patients with psychotic disorders and their family and/or carers are informed about support available to help them back into work or education, housing options, entitlement to benefits, and entitlement to drive.

If you are managing a patient with a psychotic disorder solely in primary care, NICE (2020) proposes referral to secondary care if they show a poor or partial response to treatment or treatment adherence is poor, their functioning declines significantly, they develop adverse effects from medication, you suspect co-morbid alcohol or drug misuse or if there is a potential risk to the patient or others.

Managing a relapse

If you suspect your patient is experiencing a relapse, initiate a risk assessment of harm to the patient and/or others. Refer to information regarding risk assessment above in the 'Clinical treatment and management' section (p. 110). Emsley, Chiliza and Asmal (2013) state that 'given the difficulties in identifying those at risk of relapse, the ineffectiveness of rescue medications in preventing full-blown psychotic recurrence and the potentially serious consequences, adherence and other factors predisposing to relapse should be a major focus of attention in managing schizophrenia'.

As already discussed in the previous section, NICE (2020) recommends determining the risk of harm to others by considering the patient's potential to neglect their carer responsibilities, such as parenting or providing support to others (if applicable) – this will require you to initiate local safeguarding protocols. Also consider whether your patient is a risk to the public and whether they are experiencing delusions focused on a particular individual.

For patients with a care plan or equivalent, refer to their care plan and manage their needs accordingly. It is important that you also follow the patient's advance statement where possible. If you are unsure how to proceed, seek advice from the key clinician or care coordinator stated in the crisis plan (NICE, 2020).

For patients without a care plan or equivalent, NICE (2020) recommends that if you judge your patient to be at high risk of harm to themselves or others, arrange same-day specialist assessment by the local crisis resolution and home treatment team. If they need to be admitted, every attempt should be made to persuade them to go voluntarily (NICE, 2020). However, if this is not possible, compulsory admission may be necessary under Sections 2 or 4 of the Mental Health Act. See previous chapters for more information on the Mental Health Act.

If your patient is not at immediate risk of harm to themselves or others, urgently refer them for specialist assessment. Use your clinical judgement, based on the severity of the episode, to determine whether assessment by the early intervention in psychosis service or other community mental health team is appropriate, or to determine if intervention from the local crisis resolution and home treatment team may be required (NICE, 2020).

References

American Psychiatric Association (2013). *Diagnostic and Statistical Manual of Mental Disorders (DSM-5), Fifth Edition*. Washington, DC: American Psychiatric Association Publishing, 87–120.

American Psychiatric Association (2021). What Is Schizophrenia? Available at: https://www.psychiatry.org/patients-families/schizophrenia/what-is-schizophrenia

BMJ (2015). Psychiatric assessments: how much is too much? Available at: https://www.bmj.com/content/351/bmj.h3503

BMJ Best Practice (2021). Schizophrenia. Available at: https://bestpractice.bmj.com/topics/en-us/406

Daggenvoorde T.H., Gijsman H.J. and Goossens P.J. (2018). Emergency care in case of acute psychotic and/or manic symptoms: Lived experiences of patients and their families with the first interventions of a mobile crisis team. A phenomenological study. *Perspectives in Psychiatric Care*, 54(4): 462–468.

Emsley R., Chiliza B. and Asmal L. (2013). The nature of relapse in schizophrenia. *BMC Psychiatry*, 13(50).

Gilmore J.H. (2020). Understanding What Causes Schizophrenia: A Developmental Perspective. *American Journal of Psychiatry*, 167(1): 8–10.

Harris K., Haddock G., Peters S. and Gooding P. (2020). Psychological resilience to suicidal thoughts and behaviours in people with schizophrenia diagnoses: A systematic literature review. *Psychology and Psychotherapy: Theory Research and Practice*, 93(4): 777–809.

Harrow M., Jobe T. and Faull R. (2014). Does treatment of schizophrenia with antipsychotic medications eliminate or reduce psychosis? A 20-year multi-follow-up study. *Psychological Medicine*, 44(14): 3007–3016.

Jo Y.T. et al. (2020). Diagnosing schizophrenia with network analysis and a machine learning method. *International Journal of Methods in Psychiatric Research*, 29(1): e1818.

Lieberman J.A. and First M.B. (2018). Psychotic Disorders. *New England Journal of Medicine*, 379(3): 270–280.

Margolese H.C. et al. (2004). Drug and alcohol use among patients with schizophrenia and related psychoses: levels and consequences. *Schizophrenia Research*, 67(2–3): 157–166.

Mental Health First Aid (2020). Mental health statistics. Available at: https://mhfaengland.org/mhfa-centre/research-and-evaluation/mental-health-statistics/#psychosis-and-schizophrenia

Mind (2020). Psychosis. Available at: https://www.mind.org.uk/information-support/types-of-mental-health-problems/psychosis/about-psychosis/

NHS (2021). Causes – Schizophrenia. Available at: https://www.nhs.uk/mental-health/conditions/schizophrenia/causes/

NHS England (2018). Commissioning Framework and the National Urgent and Emergency Ambulance Services Specification. Available at: https://www.england.nhs.uk/publication/commissioning-framework-and-the-national-urgent-and-emergency-ambulance-services-specification/

NICE (2011). Service User Experience in Mental Health: Improving the Experience of Care for People Using Adult NHS Mental Health Services 2011. Clinical guideline [CG136] Available at: https://www.nice.org.uk/guidance/cg136

NICE (2020). Clinical Knowledge Summaries. Psychosis and schizophrenia. Available at https://cks.nice.org.uk/psychosis-and-schizophrenia#!diagnosis

Overall J.E. and Gorham D.R. (1962). The Brief Psychiatric Rating Scale. *Psychological Reports*, 10: 799–812.

Westermann S. et al. (2020). Internet-based self-help for psychosis: Findings from a randomized controlled trial. *Journal of Consulting and Clinical Psychology*, 88(10): 937–950.

Winklbaur B. et al. (2006). Substance abuse in patients with schizophrenia. *Dialogues in Clinical Neuroscience*, 8(1): 37–43.

Bipolar Disorder

Ursula Rolfe

Case study

You are working on a double-crewed ambulance on a Wednesday evening. So far, it's been a really busy shift. You are allocated a call to attend Botham House flats to see a 32-year-old female whom you are told suffers from bipolar disorder and is feeling suicidal. Botham House is a Supported Living Project and the call has been placed by one of the support workers.

On arrival, the patient doesn't answer the door. You approach staff and obtain entry to the flat. The patient is seated on a small sofa in a dishevelled state of dress. The flat is untidy and there are overflowing ashtrays and empty take-away cartons on the floor. She asks you why you have come to see her. She states that there is nothing you can do to help her and that nobody cares anyway. She tells you she has rung the crisis team and they won't come out to see her.

Assessment

- Past medical history: 'P' was diagnosed with bipolar disorder 12 years ago when she was 18 years old. Has had several informal admissions and one detention under the Mental Health Act. P has a past history of self-harm and suicide attempts.
- Allergies: sodium valproate.
- Drug history: minor history of cannabis and regular use of alcohol.
- Social history: lives alone, infrequent contact with parents, few friends.

On Examination

- Appearance: hair unwashed or combed, casual joggers and worn-out T-shirt.
- Behaviour: staring ahead, making little eye contact. Has obviously been crying.

- Speech: slow, monotone, short one- or two-word answers initially but improves as rapport develops.
- Mood: flat in affect, seems easily distracted, lacks motivation, anhedonia, avolition.
- Thought: bleak, nihilistic, focused on the here and now.
- Perception: feels that most people and services do not care and that her family would be better off without them. No sign of paranoid ideation or psychotic symptoms.
- Cognition: concrete, black or white thinking, unable to use abstract thoughts to see any future events/possibility of change.
- Insight and judgement: has felt like this several times before and feels that she cannot keep going on like this.
- Risk: closed and guarded as to the extent of her suicidal thought and potential plans to end her own life by suicide.

Clinical observations

- Heart rate: 82 beats/min
- Blood pressure: 123/80 mmHg
- Blood glucose: 5.6 mmL/l
- Respiratory rate: 19 breaths/min
- Temperature: 36.2°C
- SpO_2: 97% on room air

Impression

P appears to be in the depressive phase of bipolar disorder and potentially experiencing suicidal ideation and intent.

Questions for consideration

1. How might the patient's presentation be different if they were in a manic phase of their illness?
2. How would you begin a conversation with P around her risk of ending her life by suicide?
3. What might be the challenges in getting mental health crisis services to respond to P in a timely manner?

Plan

Needs specialist mental health risk assessment from the crisis team but the double-crewed ambulance team needs to establish more information before they can make the referral. Key information includes:

- Any specific plans and preparation to end her own life (the more detailed the greater the level of concern).
- Access to methods, such as medication stockpile or lots of empty blister packs. (The most common method of suicide is hanging (Office for National Statistics, 2021); the most common location is patient's own home (Biddle et al., 2018)).
- Any alcohol or drug use that could lower inhibition.
- Lack of protective factors/informal support networks.
- Desire to end life, or desire to end current levels of emotional distress.
- Any recent significant events such as bereavement, bereavement via suicide, relationship breakdown, job loss, financial difficulties, etc.

It must be emphasised that no risk assessment tool will accurately predict the likelihood that the patient suffering bipolar disorder will or will not end their own life (Mulder, 2011). Research shows that around 20% of people diagnosed with bipolar disorder will end their life by suicide and between 20% and 60% will attempt to end their own life by suicide at least once (see Dome, Rihmer and Gonda, 2019).

Stephen Down

Patient voice

'During my mania, I feel like I am a god. I can do anything, so my self-confidence skyrockets. I can't explain it, but when the mania burns out, I've got nothing left. Without the highs of mania, I wouldn't be able to tolerate the lows of depression.'

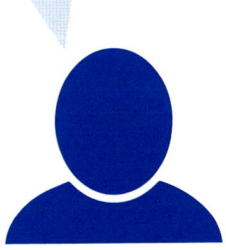

Do not do...

- If your patient is in a manic phase, don't tell them to calm down.

- Don't assume they have not taken their medication.

- Don't prescribe antidepressants if you are a paramedic prescriber – this needs to be considered by specialists in bipolar disorder.

- If you are a paramedic prescriber, do not start antipsychotic medication while awaiting specialist assessment, unless on advice from a consultant psychiatrist.

Recognising bipolar disorder

According to the Mental Health Foundation (2020), bipolar disorder is a mental health condition that involves repetitive episodes of extreme moods. Around 2% of the population have experienced symptoms of bipolar disorder which affects women and men equally (Mental Health First Aid, 2020). There are many different elements that can contribute to the development of bipolar disorder. The exact cause, like many other mental health conditions, is not known but there are a number of factors that could trigger an episode: extreme stress, overwhelming problems, genetic and chemical factors and life-changing events (NHS, 2020). Bipolar disorder may occur at any age, but it most often starts to develop between the ages of 15 and 19 and very rarely develops after 40. Research adds that recognition of bipolar disorder can take years, but most patients are diagnosed before the age of 30. The role of genetic influences in bipolar disease is supported by family studies and high concordance rates among monozygotic twins (Rush, 2003).

NHS (2020) also says that the patterns of mood swings characterised in bipolar patients vary widely. Some patients will have a few bipolar episodes in their lifetime and remain stable in between, while others may have recurring episodes with far fewer stable episodes in between.

Understanding bipolar disorder

Bipolar disorder is characterised by manic or hypomanic episodes, depressive episodes and also possibly some psychotic symptoms during the above episodes (National Institute of Mental Health, 2021). There are three types of bipolar disorder: bipolar I, bipolar II and cyclothymia (National Institute of Mental Health, 2021).

Bipolar I is characterised by having experienced at least one episode of mania: euphoria, uncontrollable excitement, irritability and agitation (confidence) that lasts at least seven days. When a patient experiences mania, they might be more active than usual, talk a lot, and very quickly, while not making total sense, be overly friendly, act inappropriately, hardly sleep, abuse drugs or alcohol, overspend and lose inhibitions (American Psychiatric Association, 2021).

Your patient may have experienced a major depressive episode, but not necessarily. Major depressive episodes are characterised by your patient losing interest in activities they used to enjoy as well as feelings of intense sadness or anger, worthlessness, guilt, fatigue and experiencing increased or decreased sleep, increased or decreased appetite, difficulty concentrating, and increased thoughts of suicide or death (American Psychiatric Association, 2021).

Bipolar II is described as a pattern of depressive episodes and hypomanic episodes but 'not the full-blown manic episodes typical of Bipolar I disorder' (National Institute of Mental Health, 2021). Hypomanic patients may show signs of being more active than usual, talking a lot and quickly, being overly friendly, hardly sleeping, overspending and losing inhibitions.

Cyclothymia is described as having experienced both hypomanic and depressive moods over the course of two years or more; however the symptoms are not severe enough to meet the criteria for bipolar I or II.

Bipolar disorder types I and II are especially difficult to diagnose accurately in clinical practice, particularly in the early stages (Phillips and Kupfer, 2013). Only 20% of patients with bipolar disorder who are experiencing a depressive episode are diagnosed with the disorder within the first year of seeking treatment (Hirschfield, Lewis and Vornik, 2003).

According to NICE (2020), you should be aware that while symptoms of depression are not needed to diagnose bipolar disorder, many patients with bipolar disorder will present with a 'depressive episode'. Differential diagnoses for bipolar disorder should also be considered, including (NICE, 2020):

- Unipolar depression
- Cyclothymia, signposted by chronic mood disturbance with periods of depression and hypomania
- Schizophrenia characterised by mania
- Delusions and hallucinations in the absence of prominent mood symptoms
- Mood disorder due to an underlying medical condition such as stroke, thyroid disease or multiple sclerosis
- Substance misuse, e.g. cocaine, MDMA (commonly known as ecstasy), or amphetamines may mimic some features of bipolar disorder.

Consider bipolar disorder if there is known drug use and if symptoms have subsided within seven days. Encouraging findings from studies with different neuroimaging modalities indicate that neuroimaging measures might help to identify biomarkers to help differentiate bipolar disorder from unipolar depression (Phillips and Kupfer, 2013).

Another differential diagnosis could be brain disease caused by dementia, cerebrovascular disease, epilepsy etc. Consider also symptoms linked to the use of antidepressants, corticosteroids, levodopa, pramipexole and prescribed stimulants such as methylphenidate. Metabolic disorders such as hyperthyroidism, Cushing's disease, Addison's disease, vitamin B12 deficiency, and renal dialysis can mimic bipolar symptoms (NICE, 2020).

Personality disorders such as borderline or histrionic personality disorder could also mimic bipolar symptoms. NICE (2020) recommends considering bipolar disorder if mood changes are rapid and do not occur in cycles. Also consider anxiety disorders, obsessive-compulsive disorder, attention deficit hyperactivity disorder (ADHD) and conduct disorder (NICE, 2020).

NICE (2020) also advises clinicians to use their judgement and to consider use of full blood counts, thyroid function tests, vitamin D deficiency and toxicology tests. They also emphasise NOT using questionnaires within the primary care remit to identify adults with bipolar disorder (NICE, 2020). In order to confirm a diagnosis of bipolar disorder a mental health assessment is needed. In order to action this, refer your patient to a specialist mental health service. Use your clinical judgement in terms of urgent referrals.

Self-help ideas for your patient

Remember that bipolar disorder can be an unsettling and difficult experience for your patient, and they may also be struggling to communicate and engage with others. It is therefore noteworthy that you can start your care of this patient with some supportive ideas to encourage their engagement in their condition. There are some tips you can suggest as well as some supportive tools which may help your patient reach out to others.

Reaching out to others

Having a support network is very beneficial. This may include family, friends or those whom your patient trusts. This network can help your patient identify when they are becoming manic or depressed and assist them in looking after themselves by listening and being understanding. Connecting with others who have similar experiences can be helpful (Mind, 2020). Contact Mind's Infoline via the website or try online community support such as Elefriends or Bipolar UK's e-Community. An analysis of online self-help forums showed that the main aim of these platforms is to share emotions and discuss daily struggles; social networking is therefore important to patients coping with bipolar disorder (Bauer et al., 2013).

Reflective practices for your patient

Mind (2020) suggests that self-care begins with the patient's understanding of their moods. Start by suggesting they monitor their moods using a mood diary. There are many freely available online. Also speak to your patient about their mood triggers. This helps in recognising patterns and then avoiding triggers or trying to lessen their impact through awareness. Suggest that the patient considers warning signs such as a change in sleeping patterns, eating patterns and/or behaviour.

Advocating a routine and sticking to it is very helpful for patients with bipolar disorder. Having a routine helps patients feel calmer if their mood is high, and motivated when their mood is low. A routine includes day-to-day activities such as specific times of when to eat and sleep, time for relaxation, hobbies and social plans and taking medication at the same time daily (Mind, 2020). Managing stress is also part of this. Encourage your patient to identify potential triggers such as finances and negative or unhealthy relationships. In fact, research shows that higher levels of stress and perceptions of less available, poor quality close relationships are associated with recurrence of bipolar disorder (Cohen et al., 2004). Therefore, advise patients to plan ahead for crises.

For many patients with bipolar disorder, insufficient sleep can trigger episodes. Getting enough sleep helps to stabilise moods and can also shorten episodes (Mind, 2020). Remind patients to eat a healthy diet and to exercise regularly.

Clinical treatment and management

According to the NHS (2020), if a patient is not treated, episodes of bipolar-related mania can last for between three and six months. NICE (2020) reiterates the importance of referral of all patients with suspected bipolar disorder to a specialist mental health service. This service will confirm the diagnosis, treat the acute episode and establish a patient-specific care plan. NICE (2020) also cautions practitioners to use their clinical judgement in terms of judging the urgency of a referral; this should be based on the results of a risk of harm assessment to the patient and/or others. Conversely, research has shown that some patients experience a significant delay in diagnosis and treatment for bipolar disorder after initiation of specialist mental healthcare, particularly those patients with a prior diagnoses of alcohol and substance misuse disorders (Patel et al., 2015).

Start by considering the risks of harm to others by assessing whether your patient is at risk of neglecting any carer responsibilities they may have (if applicable) and if this is the case, remember to initiate local safeguarding protocols (NICE, 2020). Also consider whether your patient is at risk to the public, especially if there is aggression or previous history of violence. A study by Tidemalm et al. (2015) examined the risk factors for attempted suicide in bipolar patients and found that the main clinical implication is to pay particular attention to the risk of suicidal behaviour in bipolar patients with depressive features and more severe or unstable forms of the disorder.

When determining the urgency of an admission/referral, also consider other potentially harmful consequences of poor judgement and associated actions during an acute episode that might adversely affect your patient's employment, personal relationships, and finances, and also the risks posed by driving, sexual activity, and alcohol/drug use (NICE, 2020). Refer your patient for an urgent mental health assessment if they present with mania, severe depression, or if they are a danger to themselves or other people

(NICE, 2020). Also consider that patients with bipolar disorder may be vulnerable to exploitation or violence when in an abnormal mental state. If they need to be admitted to hospital, you should make every attempt to persuade them to go voluntarily. If they refuse, compulsory admission may be necessary if they need an assessment and/or hospital-based treatment and they need admission based on their best interests and/or to protect others.

> **Remember!**
>
> Refer to the Mental Health Act 1983 for more detail regarding compulsory admission.

While awaiting specialist assessment, NICE (2020) advises clinicians not to start antipsychotic medication unless on the advice from a consultant psychiatrist. It also adds tapering antidepressant medication on specialist advice if mania develops. And finally, you should advise your patient to cease driving during the acute illness phase and that their insurance might not be valid if they continue to do so (NICE, 2020).

Your patient can be referred to secondary care if they show a poor response or adherence to treatment, if their ability to function declines, they show adverse responses to their medication, they abuse drugs and alcohol, they feel they want to stop medication after a period of stability or if they are pregnant, or planning to become pregnant (NICE, 2020).

The National Institute of Mental Health (2021) suggests that most patients with bipolar disorder can be treated using a combination of medication and psychotherapy. This can include medication to prevent episodes of mania and depression and medication that treats the main symptoms when they occur. It is empowering for your patient to learn to recognise the triggers and signs of an episode of depression or mania; suggest talking therapy and offer lifestyle advice as discussed in the self-help section of this chapter.

Medicines for bipolar disorder

Several medicines are available to help stabilise mood swings. These include SSRIs, antipsychotics, lamotrigine, lithium and valproate. (See p. 53, for further information regarding SSRIs). Other medications include second generation antipsychotics such as olanzapine, quetiapine, and risperidone (NICE, 2020). An antipsychotic may be used in monotherapy or prescribed concurrently with lithium or valproate. NICE (2020) strongly recommends that patients requiring a change in their dose of an antipsychotic or a change of drug should be referred to specialist mental health services, or that specialist advice should be sought. A systematic review by Garcia et al. (2016) examined adherence to antipsychotic medication in bipolar and schizophrenia patients and found that 'younger age, substance abuse, poor insight, cognitive impairments, low level of education, minority ethnicity, poor therapeutic alliance, experience of barriers to care, high intensity of delusional symptoms and suspiciousness, and low socioeconomic status' are the main risk factors for medication nonadherence.

Patients may be prescribed a combination of lithium and valproate if they experience rapid cycling, where they quickly change from highs to lows without a 'normal' period in between (NHS, 2020). If this does not help, they may be offered lithium on its own, or a combination of lithium, valproate and lamotrigine. In your role, as a paramedic, you would not prescribe an antidepressant unless an expert in bipolar disorder has recommended it.

Psychological treatment

The NHS (2020) suggests some patients find psychological treatment helpful when used alongside medication in between episodes of mania or depression. These psychological treatments include psychoeducation, cognitive behavioural therapy (CBT), most useful for depression and family therapy, which focuses on family relationships (such as marriage) and encourages everyone within the family or relationship to work together to improve mental health. Psychological treatment usually consists of around 16 sessions. Each session lasts an hour and takes place over a period of six to nine months (NHS, 2020). Interestingly, a systematic review by Tremain et al. (2020) examined the influence of stage of illness on functional outcomes after psychological treatment in bipolar disorder patients. Some evidence was found of an interaction between specific intervention type and stage of illness in predicting outcomes; however further research is needed to understand the impact of illness stage on the effectiveness of psychosocial interventions.

Managing a relapse

A review on predictors of relapse in bipolar disorder showed that these include 'stressful life events, increased number of previous episodes, decreased interval between episodes, and persistence of affective symptoms and episodes' (Altman et al., 2006). The authors add that factors associated with longer survival times include psychotherapy, social support, and medication adherence.

NICE (2020) advises that clinicians first assess their patient (identified as having an established diagnosis of bipolar disorder) for risk of harm to themselves and/or others. If your patient has a care plan or equivalent, ensure the care plan is followed where possible especially with reference to advance statements and crisis plans. If you are In doubt, ask for further input from the key clinician or care coordinator referred to in the patient's crisis plan. If your patient does not have a care plan or equivalent and they develop mania or severe depression and are judged to be at immediate risk of harm to themselves or others, arrange same-day specialist assessment by the local crisis resolution and home treatment team (NICE, 2020). If your patient requires hospital admission, try to encourage them to do so voluntarily. If they decline and you believe hospital admission is necessary, refer to the Mental Health Act for further information regarding compulsory admission.

If your patient develops mania or severe depression, and they are deemed not to be at immediate risk of harm to themselves or others, consider urgent referral for specialist assessment by the community mental health service, as recommended by NICE (2020). If they develop signs of hypomania or deterioration of depressive symptoms, refer your patient for a specialist assessment by the community mental health service or seek specialist advice. While waiting for this specialist assessment, do not alter or initiate treatment except on specialist advice.

References

Altman S. et al. (2006). Predictors of relapse in bipolar disorder: A review. *Journal of Psychiatric Practice*, 12(5): 269–282.

American Psychiatric Association (2021). What Is Bipolar Disorder? Available at: https://www.psychiatry.org/patients-families/bipolar-disorders/what-are-bipolar-disorders

Bauer R., Bauer M., Spiessl H. and Kagerbauer T. (2013). Cyber-support: An analysis of online self-help forums (online self-help forums in bipolar disorder). *Nordic Journal of Psychiatry*, 67(3): 185–190.

Biddle et al. (2018). Factors influencing the decision to use hanging as a method of suicide; a qualitative review. *The British Journal of Psychiatry*, 197(4): 320–325.

Cohen A.N., Hammen C., Henry R.M. and Daley S.E. (2004). Effects of stress and social support on recurrence in bipolar disorder. *Journal of Affective Disorders*, 82(1): 143–147.

Dome P., Rihmer Z. and Gonda X. (2019). Suicide Risk in Bipolar Disorder: A Brief Review. *Medicina*, 55(8): 403.

García S. et al. (2016). Adherence to Antipsychotic Medication in Bipolar Disorder and Schizophrenic Patients: A Systematic Review. *Journal of Clinical Psychopharmacology*, 36(4): 355–371.

Hirschfeld R.M., Lewis L. and Vornik L.A. (2003). Perceptions and impact of bipolar disorder: how far have we really come? Results of the national depressive and manic-depressive association 2000 survey of individuals with bipolar disorder. *Journal of Clinical Psychiatry*, 64(2): 161–174.

Mental Health Foundation (2020). Bipolar disorder. Available at: https://www.mentalhealth.org.uk/a-to-z/b/bipolar-disorder

Mental Health First Aid (2020). Mental Health Statistics. Available at https://mhfaengland.org/mhfa-centre/research-and-evaluation/mental-health-statistics/#bipolar

Mind (2020). Bipolar disorder. Available at https://www.mind.org.uk/information-support/types-of-mental-health-problems/bipolar-disorder/about-bipolar-disorder/

Mulder R. (2011). Problems with Suicide Risk Assessment. *Australian and New Zealand Journal of Psychiatry*, 45(8): 605–607.

National Institute of Mental Health (2021). Bipolar Disorder. Available at https://www.nimh.nih.gov/health/topics/bipolar-disorder/

NHS (2020). Overview – Bipolar disorder. Available at https://www.nhs.uk/conditions/bipolar-disorder/

NICE (2020). Clinical Knowledge Summaries. Bipolar disorder. Available at: https://cks.nice.org.uk/topics/bipolar-disorder/

Office for National Statistics (2021). Suicide in England and Wales: 2020 registrations. Available at: https://www.ons.gov.uk/peoplepopulationandcommunity/birthsdeathsandmarriages/deaths/bulletins/suicidesintheunitedkingdom/2020registrations

Patel R. et al. (2015). Delays before Diagnosis and Initiation of Treatment in Patients Presenting to Mental Health Services with Bipolar Disorder. *PLOS ONE*. Available at https://journals.plos.org/plosone/article?id=10.1371/journal.pone.0126530

Phillips M.L. and Kupfer D.J. (2013). Bipolar disorder diagnosis: challenges and future directions. *The Lancet*, 381(9878): 1663–1671.

Rush A.J. (2003). Toward an understanding of bipolar disorder and its origin. *Journal of Clinical Psychiatry*, 64(Suppl 6): 4–8.

Tidemalm D. et al. (2014). Attempted Suicide in Bipolar Disorder: Risk Factors in a Cohort of 6086 Patients, *PLOS ONE*. Available at: https://journals.plos.org/plosone/article?id=10.1371/journal.pone.0094097

Tremain H. et al. (2020). The influence of stage of illness on functional outcomes after psychological treatment in bipolar disorder: A systematic review. *Bipolar Disorders*, 22(7): 666–692.

Self-Harm

Ursula Rolfe

Case study

You are on a midnight shift when you are called to a 19-year-old female presenting with 'wounds'.

On arrival, you meet Sara who has a self-harm wound to her left forearm. She tells you that she has been feeling anxious with an increasingly low mood over the last few days. The wound was sustained using a clean razor blade which she had bought earlier in the day but had not been used until the last hour when the late night and a lack of social interaction culminated in an act of self-harm. She has been self-harming for the past year after a series of traumatic life experiences and feels that it helps break the tension in moments of extreme anxiety or depression. She has never self-harmed with the intent to end her life, nor has she previously sought professional counselling or therapy. She tells you that her mood is better now after the act of self-harm. The wound is of partial thickness exposing adipose tissue and gaping approximately 5 mm; it is oozing a small amount of fresh blood.

Assessment

- Past medical history: anxiety, depression.
- Allergies: no known drug allergies.
- Drug history: none.
- Social history: lives alone, smokes 7–8 cigarettes a day; alcohol intake approximately 20 units, usually drinks at weekends.

On Examination

- Appearance: Sara is dressed in trackpants and baggy jumper; she appears moderately underweight and has meticulously styled hair and makeup. She looks tired and tearful.
- Behaviour: she is behaving appropriately for the situation.
- Speech: her speech is of normal tone, rate and rhythm.

- Mood: her mood appears low, especially when she talks about her past experiences, but she is interactive and even manages a few smiles when her pet cat comes into the room to rummage through the medical bags.
- Thoughts: no formal thought disorders identified. Form, content and possession appear normal.
- Perception: appears normal.
- Cognition: there is no evidence of cognitive dysfunction.
- Affect: appropriate to context.
- Insight: she knows that she is self-harming as a coping mechanism and that there are alternatives to this. At this stage she doesn't feel that she can cope without self-harm but would be willing to explore this with formal therapy.
- Risk: denies any suicidal thoughts, is aware that she may inadvertently harm herself more significantly than intended with any future self-harm. She is future planning and does not appear to exhibit any signs of hopelessness/helplessness.

Clinical observations

- Heart rate: 92 beats/min
- Blood pressure: 108/65 mmHg
- Blood glucose: 5.2 mml/l
- Respiratory rate: 18 breaths/min
- Temperature: 36.7°C
- SpO_2: 98% on room air

Questions for consideration

- What tools are available to help risk assess this patient?
- Should sutures be avoided in this patient?
- What psychiatric follow-up, if any, should this patient receive?

Impression

Self-harm by cutting

Plan

People who have self-harmed should be treated with the same care and respect as all others. Sara should have access to clinically appropriate wound closure treatment either in the community or in the emergency department (There is no evidence to suggest that those with self-harm should not receive sutures if required – individual management of wounds should be discussed with the patient as per normal procedures). She should be offered the opportunity for immediate psychiatric triage, either through transport to an emergency department or access to a mental health crisis line if available. If she declines these, she should be referred to community mental health follow-up. Using the Australian Mental Health Triage Scale can help with this decision-making process (NICE, 2004).

Melinda (Dolly) McPherson

Patient voice

'When I cut myself, I felt no pain, just release ... but after cutting, the pain was excruciating, and I felt so ashamed and confused.'

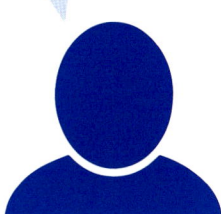

Do not do ...

- Don't be judgemental, keep an open mind about your patient and don't refer to it as 'attention seeking behaviour'.

- Don't assume someone who has self-harmed wants to die by suicide. Most often, self-harm episodes are not linked to suicide.

- Don't expect your patient to stop this behaviour even after referring them to relevant and appropriate support services.

- Don't show pity or, conversely, joke with your patient; be calm and rational in your approach.

Recognising self-harm

Self-harm refers to an intentional act of self-poisoning or self-injury, irrespective of the motivation or apparent purpose of the act, and is an expression of emotional distress. The Royal College of Psychiatrists (2020) lists the following as examples of self-harm:

- Overdose
- Cutting

- Burning
- Banging head against something hard
- Punching self
- Swallowing things that shouldn't be swallowed
- Sticking things in the body.

The majority of self-poisoning episodes involve prescribed or over-the-counter medication, and a minority involve illicit drugs, household substances, or plant material. The majority of self-injury episodes involve cutting.

Self-harm also includes suicide attempts as well as acts where little or no suicidal intent is involved (for example, where people harm themselves to reduce internal tension, communicate distress, or obtain relief from an otherwise overwhelming situation) (ONS, 2019).

The prevalence of non-suicidal self-harm has almost tripled in England over the last 10 years (Mayor, 2019). According to NICE (2020), around one in every four women aged between 16 and 24 (25.7%) reported having self-harmed at some point; more than twice the rate for men in this age group (9.7%). The rate in women aged 25–34 years was 13.2%. In addition, it is thought that the overall higher rate of suicide in men, despite the higher rate of self-harm in women, may be due to the choice of more lethal methods (firearms and hanging as opposed to cutting or poisoning). Risk factors include socioeconomic disadvantages, stress, social isolation, physical and mental health problems, drug and alcohol abuse (NICE, 2020).

Understanding self-harm

The Royal College of Psychiatrists (2021) describe self-harm as the result of a patient feeling very distressed – many patients describe self-harm as a way to release overwhelming emotions. It was also noted that some patients use self-harm as a way to express something they cannot formulate into words. Self-harm allows them to (RCPsych, 2021):

- Transform emotional pain into physical pain
- Escape traumatic memories
- Stop feeling numb or disconnected
- Punish themselves for their experiences and feelings
- Limit or reduce overwhelming thoughts or feelings
- Create a reason to care for themselves physically
- Express suicidal feelings and thoughts but without taking their own life.

A study of service providers' understanding of self-harm provided some interesting insights. Jeffrey and Warm (2009) found that 'psychiatrists and medical workers have a poorer understanding of self-harm in comparison to self-harmers and workers with psychological or social/community care training'. There needs to be an enhanced awareness and understanding of self-harm among healthcare workers so that referrals and treatments can be targeted towards individual patient needs (Jeffrey and Warm, 2009).

The Mental Health Foundation (2020) adds that the cycle of self-harm usually begins as a way to reduce a build-up of tension or pressure from distressing thoughts and feelings. Importantly, however, this provides only temporary relief from the emotional pain they are feeling because the underlying cause has not changed. The cycle thus continues with feelings of shame and guilt. The Mental Health Foundation (2020) adds that the temporary relief that some patients find at the beginning of the cycle can cause the patient to repeat the behaviour and therefore this becomes their normal way of dealing with difficult situations and feelings. It is therefore vital to talk to your patient as early as possible to help them get the appropriate support. This may not always be possible in the pre-hospital arena. Patients may need help to find new coping strategies to break this cycle, especially for long-term benefit.

Self-help ideas for your patient

Remember that self-harm can be a difficult and emotive experience for your patient, and they may also be struggling to communicate and engage with others. It is therefore noteworthy that you can start your care of this patient with some supportive ideas to encourage their engagement in their condition. There are some tips you can suggest as well as some supportive tools which may help your patient reach out to others.

Reflective practices for your patient

Identifying patterns of self-harm can help patients understand what gives them the urge to initiate their self-harm cycle. Talk with your patient and remind them that even if they are unable to resist the urge to self-harm, reflecting on it afterwards may help them gain more insight. Mind (2020) advises patients to learn to recognise their triggers; this can include situations, sensations, specific thoughts or feelings, or people. They also suggest that the patient tries to become more attuned to their urge to self-harm. Urges can include sensations such as tachycardia, anger, sadness, a sense of disconnection, repetitive or cyclical thoughts about self-harm, or making unwise decisions. Keeping a diary about these urges may help to reduce them as patients can then recognise recurring patterns.

Mind (2020) also advises that distraction may be a useful technique when experiencing the urge to self-harm. Different types of distractions work for different types of people. If your patient is feeling angry or frustrated they could try, for example, exercising, tearing something up into small pieces, shouting, dancing or shaking or hitting cushions. If they feel sad or frightened, patients could try spending time with an animal, spending time in nature, crying or sleeping, listening to soothing music, massaging their hands or wrapping themselves in a blanket. There are further examples of distraction techniques for other emotions such as feeling numb or disconnected. Your patient could try holding ice cubes, smelling something strong, a very cold shower or flicking elastic bands on their wrists. If your patient feels self-hatred and they want to punish themselves, writing poetry or songs can help as well as other creative outlets like drawing, dancing or singing (Mind, 2020).

Another self-help suggestion for your patient is to try to delay their impulse to self-harm by waiting for five minutes. Although they may not initially succeed, they should keep trying and slowly increase the delay time, building up longer gaps between the times they self-harm (Mind, 2020).

Reaching out to others

Self-help groups can also be a useful resource for patients. Research by Boyce, Munn-Giddings and Secker (2018) examined the role of these groups from the perspective of group members. They highlighted the value of self-help groups in providing opportunities for peer support and the facilitative role practitioners can play in the development of self-harm self-help groups.

Clinical treatment and management

Although treatment is always a priority, interventions for the prevention and subsequent management of self-harm should also be considered. A study on service-users' views with regard to appropriate interventions for self-harm found that there was a clear preference for specialist community-based interventions which focus on immediate aftercare while acknowledging that managing self-harm may not necessarily involve its prevention. Personal circumstances and life history are major factors in the choice of self-harm interventions. (Hume and Platt, 2007).

From a clinical management perspective, there are three pathways to consider (NICE, 2020):

- Management following acute presentation of self-harm
- Management of someone at risk of self-harm
- Longer-term management of self-harm.

Acute presentation of self-harm

This advice is based on the NICE (2020) guidelines on self-harm and considers the management and follow-up within 48 hours of your patient presenting themselves in primary care after a self-harm event.

> **Remember!**
>
> These patients may already be filled with shame and self-hatred which is why a compassionate and sensitive approach is needed.

Patients over 65 should be assessed by specialist mental health professionals; similarly, patients with moderate or severe learning disabilities should be referred to specialist disabilities teams.

Although supporting mental health is why this book has been written, in the case of self-harm patients, you also need to rule out any emergency or urgent physical injuries and treat these according to their severity. You should then assess your patient's mental and emotional state for risk factors which can include depression, suicidal ideation and misuse of alcohol, misuse of drugs, as well as gender, physical health issues, being unemployed, isolation and low financial status (NICE, 2020). A systematic review by Fliege et al. (2009) studied risk factors and correlations of deliberate self-harm behaviour and found that there were associations with current self-harm behaviour and a history of sexual abuse during childhood. Fliege et al. (2009) add that biographical stressors also play a role. As with any patients at risk, consider safeguarding procedures and referrals appropriately.

If your patient does not require referral to the emergency department, make sure you treat any wounds resulting from self-harm and consider whether to refer your patient to mental health services and don't forget to consider the needs of your patient's carers if relevant. Informed consent remains at the forefront of care provided to these patients (NICE, 2020). Make sure you assess their mental capacity if necessary referring to the Mental Capacity Act for detailed guidance.

NICE (2020) advises that you ensure your patient has access to follow-up care in primary care within 48 hours of their self-harming incident. This also includes an assessment of their risk and psychosocial needs and management of needs identified by this assessment. If possible, NICE (2020) advises preventing access to 'any means of self-harm where possible'. Consider that some patients may use prescribed drugs to self-harm. There are a wide variety of resources and support groups which patients can access via phone or online, for example, www.selfharm.co.uk; www.harmless.org.uk; www.rethink.org and www.samaritans.org. NICE (2020) advises using a multidisciplinary team approach which includes primary care and specialist mental health services. The question arises, does clinical management improve the outcomes of those who self-harm? Kapur et al. (2013) found that some patients who received psychosocial assessment had a 40% lower risk of repetition but there was little evidence that the 'apparent protective effects were mediated through referral and follow-up appointments' (Kapur et al., 2013).

Is your patient at risk of self-harm?

If your patient presents in primary care, and they are deemed to be at risk of self-harm, NICE (2020) advises that you maintain patient confidentiality. Ideally they should be seen alone and treated with a compassionate and sensitive approach as discussed in the previous section. See also the previous section for consideration of your patient's psychosocial needs and assessing these in conjunction with risk factors and safeguarding concerns. For patients who repeatedly present at risk of self-harm, make sure they do not fall through the net and are assessed thoroughly at each presentation as their risks may change dramatically with each episode of self-harm. As above, mental capacity and referral to external support systems are essential factors in the management of the patient who self-harms.

Patients with longer-term management issues relating to self-harm

NICE (2020) advises that clinicians ensure that their patients who are at risk of repeating self-harm are assessed in terms of risk, suicide and their psychological needs. Ideally, this should necessitate a referral to mental health services, but if this is not possible in a primary care arena, it needs to be completed by someone with relevant training. Refer your patient to a community mental health team if they are experiencing high levels of distress, are at increased risk of self-harm or not responding to efforts to help them and if they request specialist input. Remember that community mental health services and psychiatric liaison teams are usually responsible for the longer-term management and treatment of patients who self-harm. Their management of patients includes: helping them to stop or minimise self-harm, giving appropriate psychological interventions and creating a care plan and a crisis plan and making sure all members of the multidisciplinary team are updated about any new information. If you work in primary care, NICE (2020) adds that the role of a primary care physician includes: identifying and managing psychosocial needs, managing any other mental health issues or problems, monitoring the physical health of the patient, trying to prevent access to means of self-harm and offering advice (written or verbal) to the patient and their family/carers about sources of support and working with other relevant healthcare professions where necessary.

References

Boyce M., Munn-Giddings C. and Secker J. (2018). 'It is a safe space': self-harm self-help groups. *Mental Health Review Journal*, 23l(1): 54–63.

Fliege H., Lee J-R., Grimm A. and Klapp B.F. (2009). Risk factors and correlates of deliberate self-harm behavior: A systematic review. *Journal of Psychosomatic Research*, 66(6): 477–493.

Hume M. and Platt S. (2007). Appropriate interventions for the prevention and management of self-harm: a qualitative exploration of service-users' views. *BMC Public Health*, 7(9).

Jeffery D. and Warm A. (2002). A study of service providers' understanding of self-harm. *Journal of Mental Health*, 11(3): 295–303.

Kapur N. et al. (2013). Does Clinical Management Improve Outcomes following Self harm? Results from the Multicentre study of Self-Harm England, PLOS ONE, 8(8): e70434 Available at: https://journals.plos.org/plosone/article?id=10.1371/journal.pone.0070434

Mayor (2019). Major rise in non-suicidal self harm in England, study shows. *BMJ*, 365: l4058.

Mental Health Foundation (2020). The truth about self-harm. Available at: https://www.mentalhealth.org.uk/publications/truth-about-self-harm

Mind (2020). Self-harm. Available at: https://www.mind.org.uk/information-support/types-of-mental-health-problems/self-harm/about-self-harm/

NICE (2004). Self-harm in over 8s: short-term management and prevention of recurrence. Clinical guideline [CG16]. Available at: https://www.nice.org.uk/guidance/cg16/chapter/1-guidance

NICE (2020). Clinical Knowledge Summaries. Self-harm: Management. Available at: https://cks.nice.org.uk/topics/self-harm/management/

ONS (2019). Suicides in the UK: 2018 Registrations. Available at: https://www.ons.gov.uk/peoplepopulationandcommunity/birthsdeathsandmarriages/deaths/bulletins/suicidesintheunitedkingdom/2018registrations

Royal College of Psychiatrists (2020). Self harm. What is Self Harm? Available at: https://www.rcpsych.ac.uk/mental-health/problems-disorders/self-harm

Chapter 11

Delirium and Dementia

Carol Robertson

Case study

You are working on a falls car and at 16:00 hours, you receive a call to a 75-year-old male on the floor. His wife had requested help via her care line support (pendant). On arrival, you knock and a female voice tells you to enter. On entering the room you introduce yourself and notice a female sitting in a chair with a walking frame nearby and a man kneeling on the floor.

The woman informs you that her husband is not himself. She advises that he is her carer and this morning he brought her breakfast in bed as normal, but in the last couple of hours, he has seemed 'not quite right' and has been looking for a pill on the floor for over 30 minutes. You approach the patient and ask if you can help. You kneel at his side and ask a few questions to gain an understanding of the situation. He is conscious and breathing normally and he explains he is trying to find a tablet he has dropped; you are unable to see it on the patterned carpet but he is fixated on finding the tablet. He denies any pain or symptoms and advises you that he is fine. He agrees to sit while you assess him so you assist him to the nearest chair.

Assessment

- Past medical history: hypertension and Alzheimer's disease.
- Allergies: no known drug allergies.
- Drug history: amlodipine and donepezil.
- Social history: lives with wife, completes all activities of daily living including washing, cleaning and shopping. The house is well-kept, clean and comfortable.

On examination

- Appearance: clean, dressed appropriately.
- Behaviour: inappropriate for situation – preoccupied looking for their medication as priority, no comprehension that paramedic has entered his home.

- Speech: delayed in responses – wife reports slower in answering, quiet, monotone.
- Mood: flat, wife advised sudden change, no previous similar episodes.
- Thoughts: disorganised, fixated on finding the tablet.
- Perception: difficult to assess if hallucinating – unable to see the object he was looking for. No perception that he may cause harm to himself if not medically assessed.
- Affect: flat, lacking emotion pertaining to the situation.
- Cognition: lacks attention to questions – difficult to concentrate, as he is distracted in looking at the carpet, still searching for the tablet.
- Insights: unaware of his change in behaviour or his wife's concerns.
- Risk: does not disclose any suicidal thoughts or thoughts of harming himself or others.

Clinical observations

- Heart rate: 84 beats/min
- Blood pressure: 142/68 mmHg (lying); 145/70 mmHg (sitting); 140/68 mmHg (standing)
- Blood glucose: 7 mml/l
- Respiratory rate: 18 breaths/min
- Temperature: 38.8°C
- SpO$_2$: 98% on room air
- GCS: 14/15 (E4, V4, M6)
- Pupils: PEARL
- FAST negative
- Frailty: Mild
- NEWS2 score: 4 (ACVPU: 3, Temperature: 1)

When enquiring about his medical history he is very vague, his answers appear disorganised, and his attention is distracted as he is constantly looking at the carpet. His wife informs you that although he has received a diagnosis of Alzheimer's disease, it is mild and he functions well cognitively; however, his short-term memory can be poor. Due to his inattention and new confusion, you apply a delirium-screening tool to determine whether a possible delirium is present.

Questions for consideration

- How do you determine new confusion in a patient with a known cognitive impairment?

- How would you manage this patient?
- What would you consider the three key challenges when providing care in this situation?
- What are your safety-netting considerations for cognitively impaired patients who do not require hospital admission?

Impression

Delirium secondary to an infection due to his raised temperature.

Plan

Identify the source of the infection, determine whether the patient can be treated at home and is safe to stay at home with support. If unable to identify the cause of the delirium or arrange a supportive package, transport to emergency department for further investigation. Consider support for wife due to her carer's incapacity/absence.

Patient voice

'I would read something and forget it straight away. I got lost driving home from work on a route I had taken for years. I tried to go for a run outside my house, but I wasn't even dressed right.'

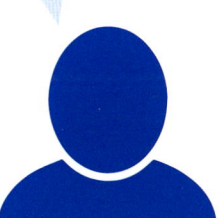

Do not do ...

- Don't engage in an argument with your patient by raising your voice or your tone.
- Don't behave in a way that could be interpreted as defensive or as doubting your patient's ability to handle a situation.
- Don't give lengthy explanations about plans or future treatments as this may cause more confusion and distress.
- Try not to question your patient's recent memory or remind them that they are forgetful.

Recognising delirium

NICE (2019) advises that delirium is also known as an 'acute confusional state'. Delirium is a symptom, not a disease and has been recognised since ancient times (Slooter, 2017). Fong et al. (2019) explain that delirium is an acute decline in cognition and attention, a familiar complication of illness, surgery, acute trauma in older adults, and is related to multiple adverse outcomes including increased disease and death. Often, delirium can lead to reduced function, loss of independence and longer hospital stays (Rahman, 2020). Some patients develop long-term cognitive decline after delirium, and delirium significantly increases the risk of incident dementia. Delirium is often unrecognised or mistaken for Alzheimer's disease (Fong et al., 2019). According to NICE (2020), the prevalence of delirium in people on medical wards in hospital is about 20% to 30%, and 10% to 50% of people having surgery develop delirium. In long-term care the prevalence is under 20%.

A patient may present with an acute, fluctuating syndrome of inattention, impaired level of consciousness, and disturbed cognition (NICE, 2020). The onset of delirium is usually over hours to days and persists for days to weeks, although longer periods have been reported (CGA Toolkit Plus, 2021). When determining the difference between a delirium and a dementia, the onset of acute changes is usually the key. For example, dementias have a gradual onset of symptoms usually over months, whereas a delirium may come on very suddenly over hours to days.

These varieties in presentations usually manifest in certain behaviours, for example, hyperactivity – increased psychomotor activity including altered perception involving vivid hallucinations, agitated, restless paranoia and aggressive manners (NICE, 2020). Patients may feel frightened or threatened by those caring for them, causing them to flee (Rahman, 2020).

Conversely, presentations of hypoactivity can hamper assessments and care due to reduced alertness and movement and/or extreme drowsiness in the patient; they may appear significantly depressed, tearful and unclear about their future (NICE, 2020). Often, thorough questioning can reveal levels of inattention and slower cognitive processing. Patients often lack interest in food and drink causing high risks of dehydration and malnutrition. They may present as an end-of-life patient (Rahman, 2020), or a mixture of all the above, which can be overlooked due to the variation in presentations (NICE, 2020).

Understanding delirium

NICE (2020) lists the following as predisposing factors where the greater the number of elements, the higher the risk of delirium. These include:

- Older age 65+ (up to 50% on hospital wards; 70–87% in ICUs and up to 30% in emergency departments)
- Having cognitive impairment
- Frailty or having multiple co-morbidities

- Major injuries

- Functional impairments

- Iatrogenic events such as catheterisation, polypharmacy or surgery

- History of or current alcohol abuse

- Visual impairments or hearing loss

- Poor nutrition

- Isolation

- In the terminal phase of illness.

Furthermore, changing environments can also have an impact on patients' increased risks; therefore when in hospital try to reduce the amount of ward changes. There are several mnemonics to help in identifying the causes of a delirium and it is worth remembering that there is frequently more than one cause.

DELIRIUMS

- **D**rugs
- **E**yes, ears, and other sensory deficits
- **L**ow O_2 states (e.g. heart attack, stroke, and pulmonary embolism)
- **I**nfection
- **R**etention (of urine or stool)
- **I**ctal state
- **U**nder-hydration/under-nutrition
- **M**etabolic or K+, Na or Electrolyte causes (DM, Post-operative)
- (**S**ubdural haematoma).

Source: adapted from SLU Geriatrics Evaluation Mnemonics and Screening (SLU GEMS, 2020)

I WATCH DEATH

- **I**nfection: HIV, sepsis, pneumonia
- **W**ithdrawal: alcohol, barbiturate, sedative-hypnotic
- **A**cute metabolic: acidosis, alkalosis, electrolyte problem, hepatic/renal failure
- **T**rauma: closed-head injury, heatstroke, post-operative, severe burns

- **C**NS pathology: abscess, haemorrhage, hydrocephalus, subdural hematoma, infection, seizures, stroke, tumours, metastases, vasculitis, encephalitis, meningitis, syphilis
- **H**ypoxia: anaemia, carbon monoxide poisoning, hypotension, Pulmonary or cardiac failure
- **D**eficiencies: vitamin B12, folate, niacin, thiamine
- **E**ndocrinopathies: hyper/hypoadrenocorticism, hyper/hypoglycaemia, myxoedema, hyperparathyroidism
- **A**cute vascular: hypertensive encephalopathy, stroke, arrhythmia, shock
- **T**oxins or drugs: prescription drugs, illicit drugs, pesticides, solvents
- **H**eavy metals: lead, manganese, mercury

Source: Wise (1986)

PINCHES ME

- **P**ain
- **I**nfection
- **N**utrition
- **C**onstipation
- **H**ydration
- **E**ndocrine + Electrolyte
- **S**troke
- **M**edication and Alcohol
- **E**nvironmental

Source: CGA Toolkit Plus 2020

When exploring a patient's medications, consideration should be given to the anticholinergics which block the neurotransmitter acetylcholine in the central and peripheral nervous systems (Moodie, 2013). These medications are often prescribed to manage a variety of conditions including depression, urinary incontinence, COPD, allergies and Parkinson's disease (King and Rabino, 2021). Older adults often have multiple co-morbidities (and therefore, multiple medications) and due to ageing processes, the ability to metabolise medications declines. Thus, older people can be more susceptible to anticholinergic effects (King and Rabino, 2021). Recent research also indicates that there is a dose-dependent association between long-term use of anticholinergics and the risk of developing dementia (CGA Toolkit Plus, 2021).

Assessment clinical treatment and management of delirium

NICE (2020) states that delirium is a clinical diagnosis based on a detailed history, examination and the relevant investigations. Taking an in-depth history from the patient and/or their advocate/observer is imperative. Ultimately, understanding the development of onset, description of events and fluctuating course of the behavioural change, is suggestive of a delirium.

Consider any precipitating factors such as acute illnesses/insult, constipation, recent discharge from hospital or fall. Systematically work through the causes mnemonic of your choice. Do not stop at the first possible source because you may find it to be multifactorial.

Check vital signs including alertness (ACVPU), temperature, blood pressure, heart rate, capillary refill time, blood glucose, ECG and pulse oximetry to assist in identifying obvious causes. These observations may lead you to consider certain conditions such as hypoglycaemia, hypoxia etc.; however, ensure a review of systems is considered.

A new presentation of confusion (ACVPU) should direct you to further assessment tools. Applying a screening tool will assist in considering a diagnosis of delirium. NICE (2020) suggests carrying out a cognitive assessment based on the *Diagnostic and Statistical Manual of Mental Disorders (DSM-5)* criteria or the short Confusion Assessment Method (CAM). The Royal College of Physicians (2019) advocates NEWS2 as a monitoring tool with the 4AT as the delirium assessment tool.

The 4AT is designed to be used by any health professional at first contact with the patient, and at any other time when delirium is suspected. It incorporates simple cognitive testing, to distinguish moderate to severe cognitive impairment, together with an assessment for delirium (MacLullich, 2014). It is not intended for repeated monitoring; however, monitoring tools such as the Single Question in Delirium (SQiD) or the National Early Warning Score 2 (NEWS2) are appropriate (MacLullich, 2014). If the monitoring tool is positive, e.g. ACVPU then utilises the 4AT for a more detailed assessment.

To help differentiate acute and chronic cognitive changes, confirmation from any medical care plans, hospital discharge letter or patient's GP may provide this information. Questions relating to their previous cerebral function and their ability to manage the home, compliance with medications, care packages and social factors may also contribute.

Identification of delirium followed by the probable underlying reversible cause of the confusional state can be a challenge. Work through the causes of delirium as a checklist, and wherever possible, ensure a probable intervention is put in place. Start with simple solutions – do they have their glasses or hearing aids? Are they in pain? Have they opened their bowels? When suspecting or diagnosing a delirium, effective communication is paramount. Ensure you are continually explaining who you are, why you are there and what you are doing. Reorientation of their surroundings may provide comfort.

NICE (2020) suggests most patients with delirium will need admission for same-day investigations and treatment.

> **Remember!**
>
> When considering what they need to take with them, do not forget their aids (walking stick, glasses, dentures), but also familiar items such as: a photo of their family, a blanket, handbag (empty of high value items), or any item which provides comfort.

However, if admission is not appropriate, targeted investigations may be required, such as urinalysis and/or a mid-stream urine (MSU), sputum culture, full blood count, folate and B12, urea and electrolytes, HbA1c, calcium, liver function tests, inflammatory markers CRP/ESR, drug levels, thyroid function tests or chest X-ray (NICE, 2020). Also, if the patient is not in their normal environment, try to create one for them.

Recovery from delirium is individual and is dependent on several factors including patient's co-morbidities, cognitive function and resilience before the delirium. Rahman (2020) highlights common outcomes following an episode of delirium, which include falls, subsyndromal delirium, cognitive impairment, 'disablement' and mortality. Death of older adults who develop a delirium during hospitalisation is nearly four times greater than those who do not develop delirium (Dharmarajan et al., 2017).

Recognising dementias

The Alzheimer's society states that (2018) 'Dementia is the UK's biggest killer. Someone develops it every three minutes and there's currently no cure'. Dementia is a life-limiting illness; however, understanding its trajectory to death is very challenging. The World Health Organization estimated that the number of people living with dementia worldwide in 2015 was 47 million and as the population ages, this is expected to rise to over 135 million by 2050 (Shi, Sabbagh and Vellas, 2020). Dementia is a cluster of signs and symptoms, which may include memory loss, problems with thinking, problem solving, perception or language; it can also affect behaviour or mood (Alzheimer's Society, 2020). It is not a natural part of ageing and is caused when diseases such as Alzheimer's or a series of strokes, impair the brain. Alzheimer's disease is the most common cause of dementia; however, there are many types including vascular, Lewy body, cognitive impairment, frontotemporal, mixed, young-onset, Creutzfeldt–Jakob disease, alcohol-related brain damage, and many less common presentations (Alzheimer's Society, 2020).

Different parts of the brain can be affected therefore producing different symptoms for individuals. Initial symptoms are usually mild; however as they progress they can affect daily life significantly. Alzheimer's disease is a sinister neurodegenerative disorder characterised by chronic and progressive cognitive decline. Pathological features include an accumulation of diffuse amyloid beta, neuritic plaques and hyper-phosphorylated tau protein in the form of neurofibrillary tangles (Shi, Sabbagh and Vellas, 2020). The pathophysiological course of Alzheimer's disease is believed to start many years (possibly decades) before a diagnosis (Sperling et al., 2011).

Vascular dementia is the second most common dementia in the UK. Within this umbrella are: stroke-related, post-stroke related, single and/or multi-infarcts, subcortical and mixed (vascular and Alzheimer's). Common presentations in the early stages include difficulty with planning or organising, making decisions or solving problems, problems following a sequence of steps such as cooking, decreased speed of thought and reduced concentration, including short periods of abrupt confusion. Patients may also experience alterations in mood; for example, they may be more emotional or demonstrate indifference, depression, anxiety or be prone to rapid mood swings, becoming either tearful or happy (Alzheimer's Society, 2020).

Understanding dementia

The Alzheimer's Society's risk factors for dementias factsheet (2016) includes advancing age (over 65) as its primary risk factor. This risk doubles approximately every five years. More women are affected; worldwide, women with dementia outnumber men 2 to 1. The exact reasons are not known, but possible explanations include that women usually live longer and it may be connected to a loss of oestrogen post-menopause.

Dementia is not usually inherited; however, this is dependent on the specific cause of the dementia. There are a minute number of families in whom Alzheimer's appears hereditary; in these few the dementia tends to be of early onset (<65 years). Older age is the biggest risk factor; evidence suggests that risk may be reduced by keeping active, eating a healthy diet and exercising the brain, especially from mid-life onwards. Pre-existing conditions such as diabetes, stroke, cardiovascular disease, hypertension, high cholesterol and obesity in mid-life present further risks while a less significant risk factor is depression. Those who have had a stroke, have diabetes or cardiovascular disease are potentially more likely to develop vascular dementia.

Clinical treatment and management

In making an initial diagnosis of dementia, it should be differentiated from depression, delirium, drug effects (anticholinergics), sensory impairments, and memory changes that are not expected as part of normal ageing (Burns, 2014). It requires confirmation of two aspects. First, that the patient's symptoms affect their daily living activities and are progressive. The second is to establish the cause of the condition (Alzheimer's disease, vascular dementia or Lewy body dementia).

NICE (2020) advocates that an initial assessment (by a non-specialist) should include: a comprehensive history (cognitive, behavioural and psychological symptoms and the impact symptoms have on their daily life) from the person with suspected dementia and where possible, someone who knows the person well. If dementia is still suspected after the initial assessment, a physical examination including appropriate blood and urine tests is required to exclude reversible causes. NICE (2018) also suggests using a validated cognitive test such as: 10-point cognitive screener (10-CS), 6-item cognitive impairment test (6CIT), 6-item screener, Memory Impairment Screen (MIS), Mini-Cog, or Test Your Memory (TYM). A normal score does not rule out dementia; therefore, referral to a specialist dementia diagnostic service for potential imaging should be considered (NICE, 2020).

Managing a patient with dementia

The aim is to support people to thrive, ensuring their physical health is managed well which may include rehabilitation for physical disabilities (Social Care Institute for Excellence, 2020). Some patients living with Alzheimer's disease or mixed dementia may have medications to temporarily ease symptoms, or slow down their advancement (NHS Inform, 2020). Medications are routinely prescribed for Alzheimer's disease but do not have benefits for vascular dementia, and are therefore not recommended. These medications are usually prescribed to patients within the mild or moderate stages and include donepezil, rivastigmine or galantamine. These medications can ease anxiety, help with memory problems, assist with attention and motivation and improve aspects of daily living. They boost some chemical messengers in the brain but do not work for everyone (Alzheimer's Society, 2020).

It is essential to understand that there can be barriers to communication. People living with dementias will deteriorate gradually. Staying physically and mentally active can help reduce the speed of deterioration (Social Care Institute for Excellence, 2020). Furthermore, consider any non-verbal signs of pain or discomfort. Scoring pain is challenging in patients with dementias, cognitive impairment or confusion. The Joint Royal Colleges Ambulance Liaison Committee (2019) advocates using behavioural cues and reiterates that no behaviour is unique to pain, but pain behaviour is unique to the person. They also suggest the Abbey Pain Score as an appropriate tool to assess pain in a patient with communication difficulties (Abbey et al., 2004).

People become progressively frail in the later stages of dementia and they may struggle to do things as they used to; however, even in these later stages, they may experience instances of clarity and some of their capabilities may return temporarily (Alzheimer's Society, 2020). Furthermore, their environment may influence how they feel, leading them to feeling comfortable and positive (Alzheimer's Society, 2020). Advanced care planning to gauge what is important to an individual is imperative.

The aim of advanced care planning is to facilitate clinical care that meets patient choices during serious and chronic ill health (Sudore et al., 2017). The document, 'My future wishes. Advance Care Planning for people with dementia in all care settings', developed by NHS England, the Alzheimer's Society and Together in Dementia Everyday (TIDE) (2018) highlights that advanced care planning is not complete following a single, isolated meeting but is an ongoing process.

Individualised care plans involve considering a person's choices, requirements and principles. Unfortunately, this can be difficult when the person lacks decision-making capacity (Gama et al., 2013). The Care Quality Commission (2016) recognises that individuals with Alzheimer's disease and frailty have poorer outcomes in the last phase of their lives than those with a single condition (e.g. cancer). They partly attribute this to the difficulty in health professionals recognising the last 12 months of life (Care Quality Commission, 2016). Therefore, as clinicians who often see patients and their families in times of crisis, it is vital that we signpost and discuss the importance of advanced care planning so that carers and health and social professionals have an understanding of the individual's wishes for their final years, months or days.

When caring for a patient in an acute setting, consideration of their normal baseline is vital in recognising when acute changes occur. Having knowledge of the common dementias enables a thorough assessment of the patient and their normal variables. Furthermore, asking if the patient has an advanced care plan, which documents the patient's baseline and their thoughts and wishes, is a vital addition when assessing and deciding on a plan of care. Consider the different systems and potential causes of your patient's delirium and attempt to rectify any obvious causes. Delirium is a medical emergency with a high mortality; therefore it is essential that clinicians do not suggest a 'worsening dementia' when there are acute changes. Any abnormal behaviours, even if accompanied by normal clinical observations, require further assessment.

References

Abbey J.A. et al. (2004). The Abbey Pain Scale – A 1-minute numerical indicator for people with late-stage dementia. *International Journal of Palliative Nursing*, 10(1): 6–13.

Alzheimer's Society (2016). Risk factors for dementia. Available at: https://www.alzheimers.org.uk/sites/default/files/pdf/factsheet_risk_factors_for_dementia.pdf

Alzheimer's Society (2018). Alzheimer's Society Strategy 2018. Who We Are. Available at: https://www.alzheimers.org.uk/about-us/who-we-are

Alzheimer's Society (2020). About Dementias. Available at: https://www.alzheimers.org.uk/about-dementia

Burns A. (2014). Diagnosing dementia: any appropriately skilled clinician can make the diagnosis and brain scanning not always needed. Available at: https://www.england.nhs.uk/2014/11/skills-to-recognise-dementia/

Care Quality Commission (2016). A different ending: Addressing inequalities in end of life care. Overview report. Available at: https://www.cqc.org.uk/sites/default/files/20160505%20CQC_EOLC_OVERVIEW_FINAL_3.pdf

CGA Toolkit Plus (2021). Delirium. Available at: https://www.cgakit.com/p-2-delirium

Dharmarajan K. et al. (2017). Pathway from Delirium to Death: Potential In-Hospital Mediators of Excess Mortality. *Journal of American Geriatric Society*, 65(5): 1026–1033.

Fong T.G. et al. (2019). Delirium and Alzheimer's Disease: A Proposed Model for Shared Pathophysiology. *International Journal of Geriatric Psychiatry*, 34(12): 781–789.

Gama A. et al. (2013). Advanced Care Planning in Alzheimer Disease. A Multidisciplinary Strategy. *European Geriatric Medicine*, 4: S120–S80.

Joint Royal Colleges Ambulance Liaison Committee, Association of Ambulance Chief Executives. (2019). 'Falls in Older Adults'. *JRCALC Clinical Guidelines*. Cited from: JRCALC Plus (2017) (Version 1.2.16) [Mobile application software]. Bridgwater: Class Publishing Ltd. Accessed September 2021.

King R. and Rabino S. (2021). ACB Calculator. [Anticholergenic Burden]. Available at: http://www.acbcalc.com/

MacLullich A. (2014). The 4AT Rapid Clinical Test for Delirium. Available at: https://www.the4at.com/

Moodie T. (2013). Anticholinergic medication. Available at: https://www.dermnetnz.org/topics/anticholinergic-medications/

NHS England (2018). My future wishes. Advance Care Planning (ACP) for people with dementia in all care settings. Document developed by NHS England, the Alzheimer's Society and Together in Dementia Everyday. Available at: https://www.england.nhs.uk/wp-content/uploads/2018/04/my-future-wishes-advance-care-planning-for-people-with-dementia.pdf

NHS Inform (2020). Alzheimer's disease. Available at: https://www.nhsinform.scot/illnesses-and-conditions/brain-nerves-and-spinal-cord/alzheimers-disease#treating-alzheimers-disease

NICE (2019). Delirium: prevention, diagnosis and management. Clinical guideline [CG103]. Available at: https://www.nice.org.uk/guidance/cg103/resources/2020-exceptional-surveillance-of-delirium-prevention-diagnosis-and-management-nice-guideline-cg103-8828117389/chapter/Surveillance-decision?tab=evidence

NICE (2020). Clinical Knowledge Summaries. Dementia. Available at: https://cks.nice.org.uk/topics/dementia/

Rahman S. (2020). *Essentials of Delirium*. London: Jessica Kingsley Publishers.

Royal College of Psychiatrists (2019). Delirium. Available at: https://www.rcpsych.ac.uk/mental-health/problems-disorders/delirium

Saint Louis University School of Medicine (2020). SLU Geriatrics Evaluation Mnemonics and Screening (SLU GEMS). Available at: https://www.slu.edu/medicine/internal-medicine/geriatric-medicine/aging-successfully/pdfs/slu-gems-book.pdf

Shi J., Sabbagh M.N. and Vellas B. (2020). Alzheimer's disease beyond amyloid: strategies for future therapeutic interventions. *BMJ*, 371: m3684. Available at: https://www.bmj.com/content/bmj/371/bmj.m3684.full.pdf

Slooter A.J.C. (2017). Delirium, what's in a name? *British Journal of Anaesthesia*, 119(2): 283–285.

Social Care Institute for Excellence (2020). Dementia: Dementia and Healthy Living. Available at: https://www.scie.org.uk/dementia/after-diagnosis/support/staying-healthy.asp

Sperling R.A. et al. (2011). Toward defining the preclinical stages of Alzheimer's disease: Recommendations from the National Institute on Aging–Alzheimer's Association workgroups on diagnostic guidelines for Alzheimer's disease. *Alzheimer's Dementia*, 7(3): 280–292.

Sudore R.L. et al. (2017). Defining Advance Care Planning for Adults: A Consensus Definition From a Multidisciplinary Delphi Panel. *Journal of Pain and Symptom Management*, 53(5): 821–832.

Wise M.G. (1986). Delirium. In R.E. Hales and S.C. Yudofsky (eds), *American Psychiatric Press Textbook of Neuropsychiatry*. Washington, DC: American Psychiatric Press: 89–103.

Acute Behavioural Disturbance

David Partlow

Case study

You are on a double-crewed ambulance when you are called to a male behaving strangely in a public place. On your arrival, an approximately 30-year-old male is found naked in the street screaming and punching the air. Police are on scene and have cleared bystanders and are moving in to restrain the patient. A police officer tells you that they have tried to verbally de-escalate the situation, but they are concerned for the patient's wellbeing as he has punched himself in the head several times and appears sweaty and unwell. It takes 6 police to restrain the patient and get him into the ambulance. You are careful to make sure that he is restrained on his back with his chest clear of any weight or restriction to breathing. As this is happening a 'friend' of the patient arrives and informs you that his name is Dan and that he took an unknown street drug 30 minutes earlier.

Assessment

- Past medical history: his friend denies knowledge of any past medical history.
- Allergies: unable to ascertain.
- Drug history: none prescribed.
- Social history: lives in shared accommodation, smoker of unknown quantity, binge drinks, regularly uses cocaine and various street and party drugs.

On Examination

- Appearance: Dan is naked, covered in bruises and abrasions. Not of large build but appears to have strength beyond his physical size.
- Behaviour: erratic, aggressive – mostly towards himself, but is actively fighting off the police; he does not interact when you try to talk to him.
- Speech: he is swearing and yelling to be let go, no obvious slurred speech or dysphasia.

- Mood: he appears angry and hyperactive.
- Thought: Dan appears to be paranoid with possible hallucinations. You are concerned about psychosis.
- Perception: his perception of the situation appears altered and he is unable to rationalise his decisions.
- Affect: irritable, hostile and labile.
- Cognition: it is impossible to fully assess his cognition but there is definitely an impairment of his cognitive functioning at this moment.
- Insight and judgement: he has no insight or judgement at this moment.
- Risk: He is currently a high risk to himself and others.

Clinical observations

- Heart rate: 160 beats/min
- Blood pressure: 204/100 mmHg
- Blood glucose: 6.0 mml/l
- Respiratory rate: 32 breaths/min
- Temperature: 39.9°C
- SpO_2: 98% on room air

Questions for consideration

1. What features make you consider an acute behavioural disturbance in this patient?
2. What risks surrounding restraint should you be aware of to prevent harm to the patient?
3. What might the in-hospital team or an enhanced skills pre-hospital team be able to do to reduce restraint time?

Impression

Acute behavioural disturbance, also known as excited delirium.

Plan

Use as little restraint as possible to prevent rhabdomyolysis, restraint asphyxia or sudden cardiac arrest. While still protecting the patient from himself, continuously assess his respiratory status while in restraint. Call for critical care backup for a rapid tranquillisation or if not possible, pre-alert the receiving hospital for earlier rapid tranquillisation for minimisation of his hyper-exertional state. Start with basic cooling measures such as the removal of clothing, place the patient in a cool environment and treat hypoxia and hypotension early. Monitor the patient closely throughout the journey (NICE, 2015; RCEM, 2016).

Melinda (Dolly) McPherson

Recognising acute behavioural disturbance

Acute behavioural disturbance or ABD may have been responsible for a number of deaths following contact with police colleagues (Angolini, 2017). It is not always appreciated quickly and can rapidly escalate in terms of clinical significance. ABD may present as:

- Unexpected physical strength
- Increase in body temperature also featuring excessive sweating or the removal of clothing
- Bizarre and/or aggressive behaviour
- Rapid breathing and increased pulse rate
- Confused thinking and speech
- Agitation, disorientation and hallucination
- Paranoia with fear of impending doom
- Insensitivity to pain.

Understanding acute behavioural disturbance

Historically, there have been a number of clinical terms used to describe such presentations, including drug-induced psychosis, excited delirium, EMD (emotionally, mentally distressed) and more recently, acute behavioural disturbance or ABD.

The Royal College of Emergency Medicine (2019) describes ABD as an umbrella term for a collection of symptoms and behaviours, although it is very important to stress that this is not of itself a mental health condition and as such, it could be asked why it is included within this text at all. It is, however, often incorrectly associated with mental ill health due to the disturbed behaviours that may be presented and as a significant clinical risk it is worthy of consideration and discussion.

The increased activity, agitation and aggression that is often seen in cases of ABD may be caused by adrenaline, stimulant drugs such as cocaine, a head injury or in some cases a mental health condition. Additionally, some medical conditions including inflammation of the brain caused by meningitis, hyperthyroidism, head injuries and low blood sugar may also be causative. Raised adrenaline levels can create the signs and symptoms associated with the presentation and increased physical activity causes spiralling acidosis. Increased physical exertion creates a need to deepen respiratory effort to increase oxygen uptake and remove carbon dioxide. The body may also produce lactic acid in response.

Anything that restricts the body's ability to increase respiratory effort reduces the body's ability to deal with the developing acidosis and that in turn creates increased risk. As detailed in the section on restraint, it is partly for this reason that prone restraint should never be used in a patient demonstrating ABD, as this significantly increases the potential to reduce the body's ability to sufficiently increase and maintain respiratory effort and can lead to multi-organ failure. Baker (2018) suggests that most cases of ABD where death has subsequently occurred were associated with a period of restraint. Baker (2018) also suggests that coroners' inquests into suspected ABD deaths have proposed that the terminology is confused and that more than 10 terms are used to describe the condition including ABD, excited delirium and autonomic hyperarousal state.

It is theorised that the increased acidosis caused by raised carbon dioxide levels in turn leads to an increase in potassium levels which can lead to cardiac arrest. Combine this with risks associated with hypoxia and it is easy to appreciate why this is considered a medical emergency. It is therefore very important to remember that anything that impacts on the body's ability to effectively maintain adequate respiration increases the risk.

An individual presenting with suspected ABD may be extremely strong and resistant, they may be paranoid or delusional and may therefore resist attempts at restraint for significant periods of time. When this is combined with stimulant drugs (which may increase the adrenergic state), or alcohol (which can bind with cocaine to prolong the effects), the risks increase significantly. Strömmer et al. (2020) suggest that sedative drugs such as marijuana may be less likely to generate behaviours which could lead to excessive methods of restraint compared to cocaine which is perhaps more likely to create a combative behaviour.

In addition, some antipsychotics can cause abnormal heart rhythm and any individual with pre-existing heart conditions such as angina or previous myocardial infarctions may have reduced capacity to withstand the increased and sustained physical activity.

Increased cardiac risk factors which may impact on the individual's ability to reduce CO_2 levels through increased respiratory effort include pre-existing respiratory disease such as asthma, COPD, and obesity. All these risk factors need to be considered in what is already likely to be a chaotic scene.

Prolonged restraint, as we have already noted, has significant potential to increase acidosis, which in turn increases the risk to life. It is important, however, to note that 'positional asphyxia' is not the only cause. Fatalities have occured even when being maintained on their side in the recovery position. As clinicians we should all be aware of the potential to occlude the supply of oxygenated blood by use of force and restraint on the neck.

Clinical treatment and management of acute behavioural disturbance

The Royal College of Emergency Medicine Best Practice Guideline (RCEM, 2016) states that ABD is a medical emergency; it reinforces the core message that restraint time should be kept to a minimum. The guidance document calls for early recognition, early intervention and for greater collaboration between emergency services on scene to ensure that clinical care is provided as early as possible.

This, in many respects is often where a joint response to an individual suspected of suffering from ABD becomes complex. Ambulance dispatch protocols are derived from triage-based algorithms and as in all areas of mental health, it is very difficult to perform triage based on an individual who cannot provide an adequate response to a triage system that feeds off binary responses. Is an individual breathing yes or no is simple; it's a closed question which when answered can support rapid determination of criticality and therefore response. While clearly a medical emergency, an individual with apparent ABD is conscious and breathing, often mobile, not bleeding or displaying signs that would trigger a binary triage process based on physical health algorithms.

Identifying ABD requires heightened clinical awareness and the ability to step outside of triage algorithms to assign an appropriate response.

On the complex, and often contentious, issue of pre-hospital sedation, the Royal College of Emergency Medicine Best Practice Guidance (2016) supports the provision of sedation, recommending that this should be managed via intravenous benzodiazepines, antipsychotics or ketamine, preferably by the intravenous route. While this is relatively simple if provided within an emergency department it is not quite so straightforward in the pre-hospital context. It is also worth adding that the provision of pre-hospital care, particularly advanced clinical practice, is not equitable across the country and the needs and challenges in delivery across urban and remote rural communities are very different and often complex. Paton et al. (2019) state that the most common rapid tranquillisation combination used in mental health services is lorazepam and haloperidol, for which randomised controlled trial evidence is very limited. Provision for rapid tranquillisation prescribing practice was not compliant with NICE guidance (NICE, 2015), which recommends intramuscular lorazepam on its own or intramuscular haloperidol combined with intramuscular promethazine.

There are significant challenges to the provision of pre-hospital sedation such as the assessment of mental capacity, the clinical competence of the clinician, maintenance of skills, legal complexities with respect to the provision of controlled substances and significant operational practicalities that create a very real challenge in terms of delivery. Maximising potential to provide pre-hospital sedation within a short timeframe necessitates a wider pool of appropriate clinicians, particularly in predominantly rural services.

With increased numbers comes greater risk with under-use of skills and therefore difficulties in the maintenance of clinical competency. Reducing the pool of appropriate staff increases the ability to maintain clinical competency but greatly reduces the ability to get an appropriately trained team on site within a given timeframe across the UK.

References

Angiolini, Rt. Hon. Dame Elish, DBE QC (2017). Report of the Independent Review of Deaths and Serious Incidents in Police Custody. Available at: https://assets.publishing.service.gov.uk/government/uploads/system/uploads/attachment_data/file/655401/Report_of_Angiolini_Review_ISBN_Accessible.pdf

Baker D. (2018). Making Sense of 'Excited Delirium' in Cases of Death after Police Contact. *Policing*, 12(4): 361–371.

NICE (2015). Violence and aggression: short-term management in mental health, health and community settings. NICE Guideline [NG10]. Available at: https://www.nice.org.uk/guidance/ng10

Paton C. et al. (2019). The pharmacological management of acute behavioural disturbance: Data from a clinical audit conducted in UK mental health services. *Journal of Psychopharmacology*, 33(4): 472–481.

RCEM (2016). Best Practice Guideline. Guidelines for the Management of Excited Delirium/Acute Behavioural Disturbance (ABD) (2016). Available at: https://www.rcem.ac.uk/docs/College%20Guidelines/5p.%20RCEM%20guidelines%20for%20management%20of%20Acute%20Behavioural%20Disturbance%20(May%202016).pdf

RCEM (2019). Faculty of Forensic and Legal Medicine, Acute behavioural disturbance (ABD): guidelines on management in police custody. Available at: https://fflm.ac.uk/wp-content/uploads/2019/05/AcuteBehaveDisturbance_Apr19-FFLM-RCEM.pdf

Strömmer E., Leith W., Zeegers M. and Freeman M. (2020). The role of restraint in fatal excited delirium: a research synthesis and pooled analysis. *Forensic Science, Medicine and Pathology*, 16(4): 680–692.

Part 3

Special Considerations

Chapter 13

Older People

Carol Robertson

Case study

You are working on a response car on a Tuesday day shift in a market town. At 12:30 you are sent to a 'pendant alarm activation' for a 78-year-old female. The only information passed is a key code to gain access and that the patient has Parkinson's disease.

On arrival, you use the key from the key safe and gain access, saying 'hello' and 'ambulance service' as you enter the property. You immediately see a pair of legs on the floor of the bedroom but no one is answering. Once in front of the patient you can see she is alert, yet appears distressed. You notice an increased breathing rate and when speaking, she is very quiet, almost mumbling her words and you notice her walking frame has fallen over.

The patient informs you that she has fallen backwards. Her speech is very quiet, flat and almost mumbling and she unable to give you much information. She denies any pain or symptoms and it is clear she just wants to get up.

Assessment

- Past medical history: Parkinson's disease, but there is no information within her apartment to give you further details. You ask about other systems, such as cardiac, respiratory and endocrine but she shakes her head to indicate there are none.

- Allergies: denies any allergies. There are no documents to confirm.

- Drug history: you are unable to confirm, as the medications are in individual, daily containers without labels.

- Social history: lives alone. There is a care file but it does not state her medical conditions or medications. It states that the patient does not mobilise without her foot calliper support. When alone, she only transfers between her chair and commode (both in the lounge). Her children attend in the morning to get her up and ready for the day, a lunch is pre-prepared for her and family visit in the evening for dinner and bedtime. Her family arrange all medications.

On examination

- Appearance: she is dressed appropriately; her hair has been brushed.
- Behaviour: appears distressed, demonstrating that she wants to get up but is unable.
- Speech: quiet, slow, mumbling, but unknown if normal.
- Mood: appears flat, but difficult to assess due to her distress.
- Thought: no formal thought disorders are identified.
- Perception: appears normal, she is aware she is on the floor and indicates that she wishes to get up.
- Cognition: slow in processing, not forthcoming with information, unknown if this is normal for the patient.
- Insight and judgement: she understands she is on the floor and wants to get up.
- Risk: She does not disclose any suicidal thoughts or thoughts of harming anyone else.

Clinical observations

- Heart rate: 72 beats/min; regular
- Blood pressure: 132/70 mmHg (lying), 136/72 mmHg (sitting, standing unsupported not possible)
- Blood glucose: 6.2 mml/l
- Respiratory rate: 28 breaths/min; once sat up, relaxed and reassured, rate 20 breaths/min
- SpO_2: 96% on room air
- Temperature: 36.7°C
- GCS: 15/15 (E4, V5, M6)
- Pupils: PEARL
- Stroke: FAST negative
- 1st NEWS2 Score: 3 (Respiratory Rate: 3)

Further assessments once in her own chair:

- Clinical Frailty Score: 7 (Severely frail)
- 4AT Delirium Score: 2 (Possible cognitive impairment).

Impression

Fall due to mobility issues. The patient states she is not normally able to walk to the bedroom alone, but she had wanted an item.

Plan

Following a full assessment of any potential injuries or medical concerns, the patient is assisted from the floor using a lifting cushion and all her clinical observations are reassessed (2nd NEWS2 score is 0). If the patient consents, a falls referral and a discussion with family (or someone who can give you a fuller understanding of the patient's normal presentation) is required to ascertain if further support is required (such as: OT/Physio/GP referrals).

Holistic Assessment: on this occasion, her daughter arrived as the patient was being raised from the floor. She informs you that her mum is acting normally but she has not had her afternoon medication for her Parkinson's disease; the daughter provides this medication immediately. The daughter also states that her mum has experienced a low mood since a stroke four years ago; however, it is undetermined if this is depression due to having reduced mobility/illnesses, or a change in her personality as a result of her previous conditions (stroke and/or Parkinson's disease). The patient also has anxiety, which often causes her to hyperventilate when she is in an uncomfortable situation (in this case, lying on the floor).

In the time it takes you to gain a full history and complete your paperwork, you notice the patient's movements, speech and general appearance are improved and you are able to now chat to her about her favourite programmes and complete a frailty screening and 4AT assessment which identifies her frailty score as 7 (looking for any changes in the last two weeks) and a 4AT delirium screen of potential cognitive impairment at 2 (Chapter 11 – Delirium and Dementia, p. 137).

The information provided by the daughter helps you to conclude that no further input or assessment is required; however, the patient would benefit from having all this rich information added to her folder or committed to a 'crisis care plan' so that information is readily available to assist any health professionals visiting when family are not available. The daughter and patient agree.

Introduction

Currently one in five adults within the UK are over the age of 65 years, which is predicted to rise to 25% of the population by 2048 (ONS, 2019). Mental health and wellbeing are just as vital in older age and it is important to remember that not everyone over the age of 65 years will have health or cognition problems. In the UK, healthy life expectancy for males is 62.9 years, and females 63.3 years (2017–2019) (ONS, 2021) indicating that for many people, ill health begins before they reach older age. Worldwide, mental and neurological disorders account for 6.6% of the total disability with approximately 15% of individuals over 60 years having a mental disorder (WHO, 2017).

What do we mean by normal ageing? It is difficult to differentiate between what is considered to be normal ageing and what are age-related variations due to the consequences of undetected disease (Fjell et al., 2014). People do not age more quickly as they get older, but what we see is an accumulation of ageing processes. The ageing process is multidimensional and can be divided into biological, psychological and sociological (Preston and Wilkinson, 2017; Dziechciaż and Filip, 2014). In 1962, Bernard Strehler (a renowned biogerontologist) defined ageing as follows:

- Cumulative: effects of ageing increase with time

- Universal: essential to occur in all species

- Intrinsic: happens internally without outside influence

- Progressive: changes leading to ageing must happen increasingly

- Deleterious: harmful to the individual

Population ageing depends on average age; therefore, improved extrinsic factors such as decreased infant death and public health involvement mean less people die in childhood or at a younger age, consequently increasing the average life expectancy. Subsequently, more people are reaching older age rather than human biology evolving to live longer (Preston and Wilkinson, 2017; Government Office for Science, 2016). Factors contributing to age-related disease include environment, earnings and education (Cannon, 2015). Furthermore, healthy ageing requires positive lifestyle choices, such as exercise and healthcare (NHS England, 2021). In addition, Kim (2009) argues that it is necessary for older adults to be actively involved in preserving their physical and mental health and that it is essential for healthcare professionals to improve older adults' beliefs about ageing. NHS England (2021) advocates frailty (instead of age) as a practical way of identifying people who may be at risk of admission to a hospital, care home or death. Conversely, Health Education England, NHS England and Skills for Health (2018) suggests in its 'Framework for Core Competencies for Frailty' that the word 'frailty' might not resonate with the public; however, it is a useful model as it aids recognition of the needs of people living with this long-term condition.

Nonetheless, frailty is not an expected part of ageing; approximately, 10% of individuals aged over 65 years have frailty, but for those over 85 years, this rises to between 25 to 50% of individuals, therefore increasing their risks of significant changes to their physical and mental wellbeing after even minor events (BGS, 2017). Those identified as living with severe frailty are at four times greater annual risk of these consequences (NHS England, 2021).

Frailty may be defined as: 'the condition of being weak and delicate' (OED). However, according to The British Geriatrics Society (2014), it is a distinctive health state related to the ageing process in which multiple body systems gradually lose their in-built reserves. Rahman (2019) describes frailty as a multifaceted state linked to multi-morbidity, disability, reliance and personal resilience.

Two globally recognised methodologies to functionalising frailty are the phenotype model and the cumulative deficit model (Rockwood, 2021). The phenotype model recognises frailty by assessing five features: self-reported exhaustion, slow gait speed, low energy expenditure, weakened grip strength and unintentional weight loss; people with no elements are classed as 'robust', one or two elements are classified as 'pre-frail' and those with three or more are considered 'frail' (Fried et al., 2001). However, the cumulative deficit model categorises frailty by considering a variety of 'deficit' features, such as diseases, disabilities, abnormal laboratory test ranges, clinical signs and symptoms (Mitnitski, Mogilner and Rockwood, 2001). Therefore, the more problems one has, the higher the probability they will be frail (Rockwood and Minitski, 2007).

The intricacies of frailty frequently go unrecognised and the multiple, interrelating social and medical issues can generate fluctuating grades of disability, therefore producing a variety of outcomes (Rockwood, 2021). Some of these intricacies are characterised as frailty syndromes which include falls, incontinence, delirium (see Chapter 11 – Delirium and Dementia, p. 137), immobility and susceptibility to the side effects of medication (Rahman, 2019; Turner, 2014), all of which are common causes of acute injury or illness in older people. Other causes are known as geriatric syndromes, which in addition to the frailty syndromes also include (while not an exhaustive list) social abandonment, sarcopenia, functional and cognitive impairment, breakdown of skin, sleep disorders and dementias (Nickel et al., 2021; Inouye et al., 2007).

Assessing an older adult

Older adults living with frailty are more susceptible to falls, immobility, incontinence, delirium and side effects of medications (Turner, 2014); furthermore, older adults with urgent care needs can suffer vital functional debility and understanding frailty helps explain why that should be so (Carpenter, Banerjee and Conroy, 2021). However, improved identification of frailty and enhanced appreciation of how to support people in living well is a key challenge for health organisations (Health Education England, NHS England and Skills for Health, 2018). Nonetheless, the benefits of identifying individuals living with frailty can aid decision making when deciding who can most benefit from support. It can assist in appreciating the impact of any insults or interventions to an individual (Moody, 2017).

As paramedics, we usually meet older people during an acute event, often out-of-hours, thereby increasing the challenges of managing patients who usually have multiple co-morbidities ranging across both physical and mental health. Therefore, this is an opportunity to think about all the ageing systems of older patients, to recognise the importance of thorough assessments and history taking, and to ask additional questions regarding their mood and interactions outside of their home. The Framework for Core Competency in Frailty helps to define the behaviours, knowledge and skills, essential to providing compassionate, holistic and high-quality care, and is contained within four domains (Health Education England, NHS England and Skills for Health, 2018):

- Domain A: understanding, identifying and assessing frailty
- Domain B: person-centred collaborative working

- Domain C: managing frailty

- Domain D: underpinning principles.

Consider an older person who has fallen. Frequent and expected questions would include: why did they fall? Were there any intrinsic or extrinsic factors? Were there any signs of syncope? The Joint Royal Colleges Ambulance Liaison Committee (JRCALC) clinical guidelines has a dedicated section on falls in the older adult that includes many aspects of assessment. Furthermore, it highlights the use of intrinsic and extrinsic factors for causes of falls; please note: mechanical fall is no longer an accepted term (JRCALC, 2021). Once you have identified the possible cause of a fall, this is not the time to stop investigating but an opportunity to consider further risk factors such as: footwear, glasses (ill-fitting slippers/socks, varifocal glasses), hydration, continence issues, skin, mood, postural hypotension, dizziness and loss of appetite. In addition, it is imperative to identify the patient's normal level of frailty and recognise any rapid deterioration that may assist you in understanding any underlying conditions (such as delirium) which might have contributed to the fall. In addition, you need to consider all aspects of the patient and investigate further injuries or illness beyond the initial disclosure of the older person. Consider some questions you might include to understand how they are feeling about growing older. Do they feel age is restricting their activities?

Many geriatricians, hospital multidisciplinary teams and community services will complete a Comprehensive Geriatric Assessment (CGA) on an older person presenting with an acute event. The CGA 'is an interdisciplinary diagnostic process to determine the medical, psychological and functional capability of someone who is frail and old. The aim is to develop a coordinated, integrated plan for treatment and long-term support' (NICE, 2016).

It is accepted that the CGA is the gold standard of holistic care with aims to generate an informed and balanced integrated care decision, considering if and how a patient may reach their prioritised and personalised goals (Buurman, Martin and Conroy, 2021). Completing a CGA is not viable in an emergency or urgent setting but having an awareness of what a CGA requires alongside conditions and the geriatric/frailty syndromes, can help develop your assessment and consultation.

> **Remember!**
>
> Always ascertain if the patient has had a sudden reduction in their physical or cognitive functions. To do this, enquire about how they were two weeks prior to today and compare the changes to aid your assessment of the acuity of changing events. You may find it useful to corroborate any changes with friends, family and/or carers which can be completed remotely (i.e. by telephone) if the patient lives alone.

As paramedics, we assess individuals on every shift and many of these patients will be over 65 years and living with frailty. Therefore, what types of questions could you ask an older person about their activities of daily living (ADLs) to aid an understanding of any changes?

Social isolation and loneliness

Older people who encounter loneliness are at higher risk of becoming physically frail (Gale, Westbury and Cooper, 2018). Social isolation and loneliness are connected with increased morbidity and mortality of older people (Roy et al., 2020).

The National Institute for Health and Care Institute (NICE) (2017) highlights the following risk factors for mental wellbeing in older adults:

- A partner has died in the past two years
- They live alone and have little opportunity to socialise
- They have recently separated or divorced
- They have recently retired (particularly if involuntarily)
- They were unemployed in later life.
- They have a low income
- They have recently experienced or developed a health problem (whether or not it led to hospital admission)
- They have had to give up driving
- They have an age-related disability
- They are aged 80 or older.

In addition, the Centre for Ageing Better and the Physiological Society (2020) recognise that the COVID-19 pandemic presented the chief risk to the health and wellbeing of older people, not just through the disease itself, but also the realisation that lockdowns placed significant restraints leading to deterioration. Their report highlights that the enforced isolation led to 32% of older people having reduced physical activity during the first lockdown with almost half citing they had no motive or less purpose to be active (Centre for Ageing Better and the Physiological Society, 2020). More disturbing are the clinical and health risks associated with reduced physical activity such as the decline in muscle protein due to reduced activity, loss of muscle mass, development of insulin resistance and metabolic inflexibility, loss of cardio-respiratory fitness and increase in body fat due to consumption of energy in excess of requirements (Centre for Better Ageing and the Physiological Society, 2020). If you consider this clinical picture alongside an older adult living with frailty, the connection between the increased risk of immobility and falls becomes apparent, therefore potentially leading to poorer mobility and increased dependence, which in turn is associated with poorer mental wellbeing (Centre for Ageing Better and the Physiological Society, 2020; NICE, 2015).

The Local Government Association and Association of Directors of Public Health have produced advice for councils to help them tackle the repercussions of loneliness and social isolation because of COVID-19. They advise this is a 'serious public health concern', leading to an increase in premature deaths similar to those associated with smoking and alcohol consumption. It is also a greater risk for developing depression (The Local Government Association and Association of Directors of Public Health, 2020). Many lonely individuals are known to the health and social care systems due to their high intensity use of services; however, there are many who suffer in silence. Worryingly, many older people are less likely to seek professional support when they encounter challenges relating to their mental health (Reynolds et al., 2020).

Common reasons for older adults to contemplate suicide include bereavement, estrangement from families, relationships and social support and risk of functional impairment associated with poor health (Conwell, Van Orden and Caine, 2011).

What questions could you ask your patient when looking for signs of loneliness, physical or mental ill-health? What could you consider doing to help a patient in these circumstances?

Capacity

As Rahman (2019) states, 'the ageing brain is characterised by structural and functional changes to microglial cells'. However, an unwell older patient who has frailty, does not necessarily lack capacity (British Geriatrics Society, 2019). Capacity is assumed to be present until shown not to be and an important aspect in decision making is the needs and wishes of the patient (Mental Capacity Act, 2005; Nickel et al., 2021). For those older adults who have decision-making capacity, even if they have an advance statement, an Advance Decision to Refuse Treatment (ADRT) or a Lasting Power of Attorney (LPA), it is still necessary to discuss options of care incorporating their wishes and goals. Many older people will want to retain their independence within their own environment (Snyder and Shah, 2016). For those patients who require assessment, the test must be specific to the decision in question, and can be completed by any professional with appropriate training (British Geriatrics Society, 2019). The Mental Capacity Act is intended to safeguard and enable people to make their own choices about their care and applies to people aged 16 and over (NHS, 2021). The Mental Capacity Act enables decisions in all areas of an individual's life, from shopping to moving into a care facility (NHS, 2021).

The British Geriatrics Society (2019) suggests two stages in the testing of capacity:

1. 'The patient cannot make a decision due to "a condition of mind or brain." For older people this is most often dementia or delirium, but other conditions such as learning disability or severe depression may also occur. It therefore follows that if a person does NOT have a condition of mind or brain, capacity should be assumed present.'

2. 'The person cannot understand, retain, weigh up, or communicate information relevant to the decision in question. Evidence of inability to do this relevant to the decision must be recorded.'

When an individual lacks capacity, consideration of any formal statements (ADRT or LPA for health) should be reviewed to ensure care is in line with their wishes.

The challenge is the patient who lacks capacity and does not hold any documented plans; but it is an opportunity (ensuring confidentiality) to discover the person's wishes including their views, principles and preferences by discussing with others (Nickel et al., 2021). Advanced care planning for those who do not demonstrate capacity should consider the patient's prior wishes and be completed with the best interest of the patient at the forefront (British Geriatrics Society, 2019; NHS England, 2018). The 'My Future Wishes' document recommends still involving the person in the care planning process as well as possibly an Independent Mental Capacity Advocate (NHS England, 2018). However, it is essential to clearly document any decision-making assessments when deciding that an individual lacks capacity (BGS, 2019).

Safeguarding

Older adults can be vulnerable to many forms of abuse including physical, psychological, material, institutional, sexual and domestic, as well as financial exploitation, discrimination, modern slavery, abandonment, neglect (active and passive) and self-neglect (Nickel et al., 2021; Age UK, 2020; Snyder and Shah, 2016). All individuals have the right to live without harm and the Care Act 2014 and the Social Services and Wellbeing Act (Wales) 2014 sets out the legal framework for all organisations to adhere to (Office of the Public Guardian, 2019).

Always be alert to evidence of potential abuse. Your presence in someone's home may be the only time a maltreated older adult sees another person or has an opportunity to leave their home or the institution (Nickel et al., 2021). The ageing population puts more strain on carers and the systems in place for care of older people so good observational skills are essential. Abuse of older people often differs from that seen in younger people (Pilbery, 2013). Furthermore, research suggests victims more frequently seek urgent care for acute illness and are less likely to have routine appointments (Nickel et al., 2021). In addition, many older adults may be facing, or at risk of, more than one type of neglect or abuse, including fraud (Age UK, 2020). Individuals at 85 years are a higher risk of a safeguarding enquiry (Age UK, 2020). Lastly, when visiting an older person be suspicious of new, unidentified individuals. If you notice a home becoming sparse of valuable possessions, this could indicate the person is a victim of 'cuckooing' (Salford Safeguarding Adult Board, 2021). The homes of vulnerable adults are often targeted. This is when criminals and their associates move into the person's property and gain control, so they can use the home as a base for criminal activities (Salford Safeguarding Adult Board, 2021).

Support and interventions for older people

To enable you to support older adults, whether during an acute event or when caring for an ageing relative, there are many resources available. Most local authorities will have a section on their website, signposting individuals to where and how they can request a social needs assessment to determine what care is available and whether the individual meets the criteria for inclusion. In addition, many general practitioners have social prescribers who can assist in helping to meet an individual's needs, whether that is help with walking a dog or a befriending service. Below are many common websites and phone lines that may assist with caring for older people.

- Age UK Advice line: 0800 678 1602. Lines are open 08.00–19.00, 365 days a year at https://www.ageuk.org.uk/services/age-uk-advice-line/

- Age UK befriending services at https://www.ageuk.org.uk/services/befriending-services/

- Age UK at https://www.ageuk.org.uk/

- British Red Cross: This organisation can assist with loneliness, financial advice and support, loan commodes or wheelchairs, locate missing family, provide assistance to stay at home (transport home from hospital, door-to-door transport for essential healthcare journeys), help with everyday tasks (collecting prescriptions and shopping), companionship and rebuilding confidence. https://www.redcross.org.uk/get-help/get-support-at-home.

- Dementia UK Helpline: 0800 888 6678 and at https://www.dementiauk.org/contact-us-details/

- Lunch clubs – usually available on council and/or local Facebook group websites.

- Parkinson's UK Helpline 0808 800 0303: and at https://www.parkinsons.org.uk/

- Royal Voluntary Service (RVS): 0808 196 3646 0800-2000. The RVS provide assistance with collecting shopping, medication or other essential supplies. https://www.royalvoluntaryservice.org.uk/our services/social-activities

- Silverline is a helpline for older people: 0800 4 70 80 9 and at https://www.thesilverline.org.uk/what-we-do/

- Social prescribers: available via GP or local authority websites.

- University of the Third Age (U3A). UK-wide movement of locally-run interest groups that provide a wide range of opportunities to come together to learn for fun. Members explore new ideas, skills and activities together. https://www.u3a.org.uk/about

References

AGE UK (2020). Factsheet 78. Safeguarding older people from abuse and neglect. Available at: https://www.ageuk.org.uk/globalassets/age-uk/documents/factsheets/fs78_safeguarding_older_people_from_abuse_fcs.pdf

British Geriatrics Society (2014). Fit for Frailty Part 1: Consensus best practice guidance for the care of older people living in community and outpatient settings. Available at: https://www.bgs.org.uk/sites/default/files/content/resources/files/2018-05-23/fff_full.pdf

British Geriatrics Society (2019). 15. CGA in Primary Care Settings: Mental capacity issues. Available at: https://www.bgs.org.uk/resources/15-cga-in-primary-care-settings-mental-capacity-issues

Buurman B., Martin F. and Conroy S. (eds) (2021). Silver Book II: Holistic assessment of older people. Available at: https://www.bgs.org.uk/resources/silver-book-ii-holistic-assessment-of-older-people

Cannon M.L. (2015). What is aging? *Disease-a-Month*, 61(11): 454–459.

Carpenter C., Banerjee J. and Conroy S. (2021). Silver Book II: Foreword and Introduction. Available at: https://www.bgs.org.uk/resources/silver-book-ii-foreword-and-introduction

Centre for Ageing Better and the Physiological Society (2020). A National COVID-19 Resilience Programme: Improving the health and wellbeing of older people during the pandemic. Available at: https://www.physoc.org/policy/covid19resilience/

Conwell Y., Van Orden K. and Caine E.D. (2011). Suicide in Older Adults. *Psychiatric Clinics of North America*, 34(2): 451–468.

Dziechciaż M. and Filip R. (2014). Biological psychological and social determinants of old age: Bio-psycho-social aspects of human aging. Annals of Agricultural and Environmental Medicine. *Annals of Agricultural and Environmental Medicine*, 21(4): 835–838.

Fjell A.M. et al. (2014). What is normal in normal aging? Effects of aging, amyloid and Alzheimer's disease on the cerebral cortex and the hippocampus. *Progress in Neurobiology*, 117: 20–40.

Fried L.P. et al. (2001). Frailty in older adults: evidence for a phenotype. *The Journals of Gerontology Series A.*, 56(3): 146–156.

Gale C.R., Westbury L. and Cooper C. (2018). Social isolation and loneliness as risk factors for the progression of frailty: the English Longitudinal Study of Ageing. *Age and Ageing*, 47(3): 392–397.

Government Office for Science. (2016). *Future of an Ageing Population*. Available at: https://assets.publishing.service.gov.uk/government/uploads/system/uploads/attachment_data/file/535187/gs-16-10-future-of-an-ageing-population.pdf

Health Education England, NHS England and Skills for Health (2018). Framework for Core Competencies for Frailty. Available at: https://skillsforhealth.org.uk/info-hub/frailty-2018/

Inouye S.K., Studenski S., Tinetti M.E. and Kuchel G.A. (2007). Geriatric syndromes: clinical, research, and policy implications of a core geriatric concept. *Journal of the American Geriatric Society*, 55(5): 780–791.

Joint Royal Colleges Ambulance Liaison Committee, Association of Ambulance Chief Executives. (2019). 'Falls in Older Adults'. *JRCALC Clinical Guidelines*. Cited from: JRCALC Plus (2017) (Version 1.2.16) [Mobile application software]. Bridgwater: Class Publishing Ltd. Accessed September 2021.

Kim S.U. (2009). Older people's expectations regarding ageing, health-promoting behaviour and health status. *Journal of Advanced Nursing*, 65(1): 84–91.

Local Government Association and Association of Directors of Public Health (2020). Loneliness, social isolation and COVID-19. Available at: https://local.gov.uk/loneliness-social-isolation-and-covid-19#_edn1

Mental Capacity Act (2005) Legislation. Available at: https://www.legislation.gov.uk/ukpga/2005/9/section/1

Mitnitski A.B., Mogilner A.J. and Rockwood K. (2001). Accumulation of deficits as a proxy measure of aging. *Scientific World Journal*, 1: 323–36.

Moody D. (2017). 'Finding Frailty' System benefits of frailty identification. Presented at: NHS England, The 3rd National Frailty Conference, Leeds. Available at: https://static1.squarespace.com/static/5b5f1d4e9d5abb9699cb8a75/t/5b911645562fa7cd9913a6b4/1536235082006/moody_finding_frailty.pdf

NHS England (2021). Ageing well and supporting people living with frailty. Available at: https://www.england.nhs.uk/ourwork/clinical-policy/older-people/frailty/

NICE (2015). Older people: independence and mental wellbeing. NICE guideline [NG32]. Available at: https://www.nice.org.uk/guidance/ng32/resources/older-people-independence-and-mental-wellbeing-pdf-1837389003973

NICE (2016). Transition between inpatient hospital settings and community or care home settings for adults with social care needs. Quality standard [QS136]. Available at: https://www.nice.org.uk/guidance/qs136/resources/transition-between-inpatient-hospital-settings-and-community-or-care-home-settings-for-adults-with-social-care-needs-pdf-75545422401733

NICE (2017). Parkinson's disease in adults: diagnosis and management. NICE guideline [NG71]. Available at: https://www.nice.org.uk/guidance/ng71/evidence/full-guideline-pdf-4538466253

Nickel C., Arendts G., Lucke J. and Mooijaart S. (eds) (2021). Geriatric syndromes. Principal Projection – UK population in age groups, 2018-based edition. Available at: https://www.ons.gov.uk/peoplepopulationandcommunity/populationandmigration/populationprojections/datasets/tablea21principalprojectionukpopulationinagegroups

ONS (2021). Health state life expectancies, UK: 2017 to 2019. Available at: https://www.ons.gov.uk/peoplepopulationandcommunity/healthandsocialcare/healthandlifeexpectancies/bulletins/healthstatelifeexpectanciesuk/2017to2019

Office of the Public Guardian (2019) Policy paper. Safeguarding strategy 2019 to 2025: Office of the Public Guardian. Available at: https://www.gov.uk/government/publications/safeguarding-strategy-2019-to-2025-office-of-the-public-guardian/safeguarding-strategy-2019-to-2025-office-of-the-public-guardian

Parkinson's UK (2019a). Types of Parkinsonism. Available at: https://www.parkinsons.org.uk/information-and-support/types-parkinsonism

Parkinson's UK (2019b). 'Get It On Time': The case for improving medication management for Parkinson's. Available at: https://www.parkinsons.org.uk/sites/default/files/2019-10/CS3380%20Get%20it%20on%20Time%20Report%20A4%20final%2026.09.2019-compressed%20%281%29.pdf

Pilbery R. (eds) (2013). *Nancy Caroline's Emergency Care in the Streets, 7th Edition.* Burlington, MA: Jones and Bartlett Learning.

Rahman S. (2019). *Living with Frailty: From Assets and Deficits to Resilience.* Abingdon: Routledge.

Reynolds K. et al. (2020). Older Adults' Narratives of Seeking Mental Health Treatment: Making Sense of Mental Health Challenges and 'Muddling Through' to Care. *Qualitative Health Research*, 30(10): 1517–1528.

Rockwood K. (2021). Silver Book II: Frailty. Available at: https://www.bgs.org.uk/resources/silver-book-ii-frailty

Rockwood K. and Mitnitski A. (2007). Frailty in relation to the accumulation of deficits. *Journals of Gerontology, Series A: Biological Sciences and Medical Sciences*, 62(7): 722–727.

Roy J. et al. (2020). COVID-19 in the geriatric population. *International Journal of Geriatric Psychiatry*, COVID-19 Special Issue, 35(12): 1437–1441.

Salford Safeguarding Adult Board (2021). Cuckooing. Available at: https://safeguardingadults.salford.gov.uk/guidance-pages/cuckooing/

Snyder D.R. and Shah M.N. (eds) (2016). *Geriatric Education for Emergency Medical Services, 2nd Edition.* Burlington, MA: Jones and Bartlett Learning.

Strehler B. (1962). *Time, Cells and Aging.* New York and London: Academic Press.

Temlett J. and Thompson P. (2006). Reasons to admission for hospital for Parkinson's disease. *Internal Medicine Journal*, 36(8): 524–526.

Turner G. (2014). Recognising Frailty. Available at: https://www.bgs.org.uk/resources/recognising-frailty

Wilkinson I. and Preston J. (2017). 4.01 Theories of Ageing. The Hearing Aid Podcasts. [Podcast]. Available at: http://thehearingaidpodcasts.org.uk/episode-4-01-theories-of-ageing/

World Health Organization (2017). Mental health of older adults. Available at: https://www.who.int/news-room/fact-sheets/detail/mental-health-of-older-adults

Children and Young People

Chapter 14

Will Murcott

Case study

You are working as a paramedic on a double crewed ambulance. Your next job comes in and you are dispatched to a 13-year-old female who was discovered by her father, locked in their bathroom, emptying cans of aerosol.

The patient had been out that evening with her family (minus mum) to celebrate her 13th birthday. According to dad the evening had gone well. After arriving back home the patient's sibling noticed aerosol gas coming from under the bathroom door. When dad forced the door open and asked the patient what she was doing she said she was trying to 'gas' herself.

On arrival the patient is very reluctant to speak to you. She is refusing to make eye contact or answer any questions. Dad is very distressed and mum is reported to be in bed.

Assessment

- Past medical history: no significant past medical history
- Allergies: no known allergies
- Drug history: none
- Social history: patient attends secondary school. No issues of bullying have been reported and the patient regularly attends drama club. Patient has two younger siblings, father who is in full-time employment and mother who is diagnosed with bipolar disorder which is not well-maintained. Both parents live in the same home.

To build rapport with the patient you decide to ask her about her interests and what she enjoys doing, while your crewmate takes dad aside to gain a more detailed history. Dad reports that he was not aware of his daughter self-harming. However recently she has taken to wandering off on her own and on one occasion he had found her stood on the edge of a bridge.

After 10 minutes you are able to get the patient to open up. She starts to answer questions about what has happened although most of her responses are limited to 'I don't know what I was thinking'.

On examination

- Appearance: the patient is dressed in jeans and a hoodie which appear clean and well fitted. The patient has a healthy pallor. She also does not appear over- or underweight for her age.
- Behaviour: initially the patient refuses to answer your questions limiting her responses to 'I don't know'. At first you find it difficult to gauge whether the patient is embarrassed or upset or whether she is trying to obstruct the assessment. When the patient does start to engage, eye contact improves and she starts to show more genuine facial expressions such as smiling.
- Speech: normal, no slurring to suggest poisoning or intoxication.
- Mood: the patient appears low in mood and detached. Not knowing the patient makes it difficult to assess how much of this was due to natural shyness or teenage 'awkwardness' or the result of deteriorating mental health.
- Thoughts: no formal thought disorders identified.
- Perception: it is possible the patient has a lack of perception. Given what the patient was found doing and her comment that she was trying to gas herself there is a strong probability that she was trying to intentionally self-harm and understood the consequences of this. However, given her age there is also a possibility that she lacked perception and did not fully understand the consequences of what she was doing.
- Affect: unknown
- Cognition: this appears intact, no reports of any learning disability.
- Insight and judgement: this appears lacking. When you describe the harm that could result from aerosol inhalation the patient simply shrugs her shoulders. In addition to this she does not provide any further insight into why she had been found standing on the edge of a bridge.
- Risk: the patient is non-committal when asked whether she wants to end her life and as mentioned above was unable to provide further insight as to why she had been found standing on the edge of a bridge. The only thing she was emphatic about is that, when asked, she said she was not being bullied and she has friends. Father confirmed that she does meet up with friends and socialises outside of school. A further risk was the mother's current mental health status and that this was apparently not well-maintained.

Clinical Observations

- Heart rate: 95 beats/min
- Blood pressure: 104/67 mmHg
- Blood glucose: 5.4 mml/l

- Respiratory rate: 18 breaths/min
- Temperature: 36.7°C
- SpO$_2$: 100% on room air

Questions for consideration

1. What tools might you use to encourage the patient to open up about how she is feeling?
2. When the patient refused to talk what are the challenges to your assessment and how do you overcome this?
3. How would you manage this situation if the patient refused to talk to you and then refused to attend ED, taking into consideration her age? How would you safety net this situation?
4. What advice would you give to the patient's father to help manage this situation moving forward? What additional referrals or signposting to other services might you offer?

Impression

Suicidal ideation due to unknown cause. Patient also displaying some behaviours which may come from a desire for increased attention, possibly due to family situation and impact of mother's mental health.

Plan

You decide that the patient requires a mental health crisis intervention; however she initially refuses to attend the local ED. The out of hours GP service is contacted for further advice despite dad stating he would be fine managing his daughter at home. The GP is concerned about discharging the patient at home and reiterated that the patient should attend ED. You renegotiate with the patient and manage to persuade her to attend ED. Once handing the patient over at ED, after consulting with the patient and her father and gaining their consent, you complete a safeguarding children's referral.

Safeguarding considerations in context of case study

This case study highlights the importance of a number of considerations in relation to safeguarding young people in the emergency care setting. Primarily it is about building rapport and trust quickly with the patient to enable them to feel comfortable about disclosing personal feelings relating to their mental state. Paramedics often feel under pressure when arriving on scene to assess, treat and then handover or discharge a patient before moving on to the next incident. When it comes to those experiencing a mental health crisis (particularly young people) it is essential that appropriate time is given to ensure a patient feels that they are being listened to and the best possible plan is devised to deal with their crisis.

Secondly, when dealing with a young person in mental health crisis and displaying suicidal ideation, appropriate safety netting must be put in place. Despite the father in the case study saying he would be fine dealing with this situation, the paramedic was concerned that once they left, the situation would escalate again resulting in the patient causing themselves significant harm. Given the patient's current and historical behaviour, as well as family environment, the paramedic felt the patient and her family required additional support moving forward, hence completing a safeguarding referral. Wherever possible a person-centred approach should be taken when completing a safeguarding referral and every step should be taken to gain child and parental consent. In addition to this it is essential that paramedics follow the principles of the Children's Act 1989 and 2004 which states that the welfare of a child should be paramount and that, wherever reasonably possible, parents should be supported to play a full part in their lives (HM Government, 2018).

Dealing with someone in mental health crisis can rarely be resolved through one, time-limited intervention like setting a leg in plaster or stitching a wound. A holistic approach is essential which is why a safeguarding referral is so important in a situation such as this to bring the relevant partners together. In doing so a paramedic can support someone to start promoting their own mental health and wellbeing and reduce their reliance on emergency services.

James Field

Introduction

Recognition for the mental wellbeing of children and young people has never been as high profile as it has in recent years. It is estimated that one in seven young people meet the diagnostic criteria for a mental disorder (Polanczyk et al., 2015). The World Health Organization identified child and adolescent mental health as a global public health concern (WHO 2014; WHO, 2020), stating that 16% of the global burden of disease for people aged 10 to 19 years was from mental health conditions. Because of the impact of this on the world's young population it is thought that this poses the largest threat to social and economic development that a country could face (McGorry, 2017).

Mental health in children

Although childhood can be a time for development, experimentation, learning, play and growth, a child could face many challenges. Epidemiological studies indicate that childhood is where it is most likely that mental health problems will begin, with half of all mental health conditions starting by 14 years, and three-quarters by 25 years (Kessler, Amminger and Aguilar-Gaxiola, 2007; Jones, 2013). In high-income countries such as the UK, mental ill-health is responsible for the highest burden of disease for people aged 0 to 25 years (Erskine et al., 2015). What this tells us is that young people are facing significant adversity and challenges to their development which can then further affect their life-course as adults. Of key importance to those working in pre-hospital care is the knowledge that despite children and young people having higher risk and prevalence of mental ill-health, they are undertreated by professional services; less than two-thirds of young people with mental health problems and their families access any professional help (Sadler et al., 2018). The pathways that children and young people take in order to access services can be fraught with multiple help-seeking attempts and lengthy delays. Typically, primary care settings play a large role in pathways for care, but there is a notable use of emergency hospitalisations and high rates of emergency services involvement (MacDonald et al., 2018). It is not fully understood why this is the case, but barriers to young people's help-seeking include societal views and attitudes towards mental health; lack of knowledge and self-reliance may also be factors in reduced help-seeking (Radez et al., 2021).

In the UK there are now more children admitted to hospital for mental health than medical reasons (Turner, 2021), and correlating with this is an increase in the attendance at emergency departments (ED) for children and young people under the age of 20. Currently, these attendances make up around a quarter of all attendances per year but the number is expected to rise by 50% by 2030 (RCPCH, 2019). What has been observed is a doubling in recent years in ED attendance by young people with a mental health condition. Alongside the help-seeking barriers previously mentioned, there are also concerns regarding the suitability and ability of child and adolescent mental health services to manage the current demand (Young, 2018). Less is known about the route that children and young people take to ED, but it is thought that ambulance call-outs for children with mental health problems are rising (Joseph, 2018). Gadancheva, Barry and McNicholas (2019) noted that for children and young people who attended ED many, roughly a third, will be first time presentations and will not be known to mental health services. What the above indicates is that it is becoming increasingly common that children and young people are presenting to ED for their mental health needs, that it is likely that it could be their first contact with services and that they may contact emergency services to do this.

Why young people go to emergency departments

Suicide and self-harm are the leading causes of death for boys and girls aged 5–19 (ONS, 2015) and young adults, both men and women aged 20–34 (ONS, 2020). With self-harm increasing the likelihood that a person will complete suicide by 50 to 100 times, it is therefore of considerable importance to ensure that young people who self-harm are taken seriously and cared for appropriately (Hawton et al., 2003; Owens, Horrocks and House, 2002). Presentations for self-harm have increased over the years, and it is thought to affect around one in five to ten young people (Wadman et al., 2020), but because self-harm is secretive and stigmatised this is probably a significant underestimate of the true picture (Clements et al., 2016). It is likely that ambulance staff will come into contact with young people who self-harm as the rates of attendance for children who self-harm are increasing. This is comparable to young people who attend ED and have a psychiatric diagnosis; for instance in 2017–18, the numbers of ED attendances for children with psychiatric conditions and children who self-harmed were around 27,000 and 22,000 respectively (Young, 2018).

Concerns for the mental health of children have been notable on several fronts. From a medical perspective, epidemiological data indicates that most, three-quarters, of mental health disorders will begin before the age of 25 years and half before the late teens. It is yet to be fully understood why this might be the case, but indications point to factors including developmental transitions, social determinants for health and wellbeing, genetic factors and environmental factors. Unique among these are developmental factors that a child or young person must navigate, some which will be explored shortly.

Legal aspects

Working with children and young people requires an understanding of the legal issues that relate to people under 18 years old. Key legal concepts when working in healthcare are consent and capacity, and both have differences to how these are understood when working with adults over 18 years old.

In short, when gaining consent from a person under 18, it is imperative that it is known whether the person is under the age of 16. If the child is between 16 and 18, the Family Law Reform Act 1969 empowers the person to consent for themselves in matters of medical, surgical or dental treatment and the Mental Capacity Act 2005 makes the assumption that they are competent to do so unless proven otherwise. A person between 16–18 years can therefore consent to, but not refuse, treatment and refusal can be overridden by a person who has parental responsibility.

If a person is under 16 years old the presumption in law is that they are not competent to make a decision and that parents, or a person with parental responsibility can consent on the child's behalf. The outcome of the court's decision made in *Gillick* v. *West Norfolk & Wisbech Area Health Authority* [1986] held that there was no automatic right for a child under 16 to be able to consent, but where a child can be assessed as able to comprehend the full ramifications of the decision then they can make the decision on their own behalf (Avery, 2017). A child who can demonstrate the necessary competence is often deemed as being 'Gillick competent', the following aspects of which are necessary, that is, the child:

- Understands the nature and degree of their condition
- Understands what is being proposed
- Understands the complications or side effects
- Understands the expected outcome, and the consequences of not having the treatment
- Is able to make a decision based on the above (Cornock, 2015).

Only adults over 18 years old who are competent have the legal right to consent and refuse treatment on their own behalf. What this means in practice is that a refusal of treatment for any person under 18 is not legally valid as it can be overridden by someone who has parental responsibility or a court. A brief summary adapted from Avery (2017) provides a flow chart to address the decision making for children (Figure 14.1).

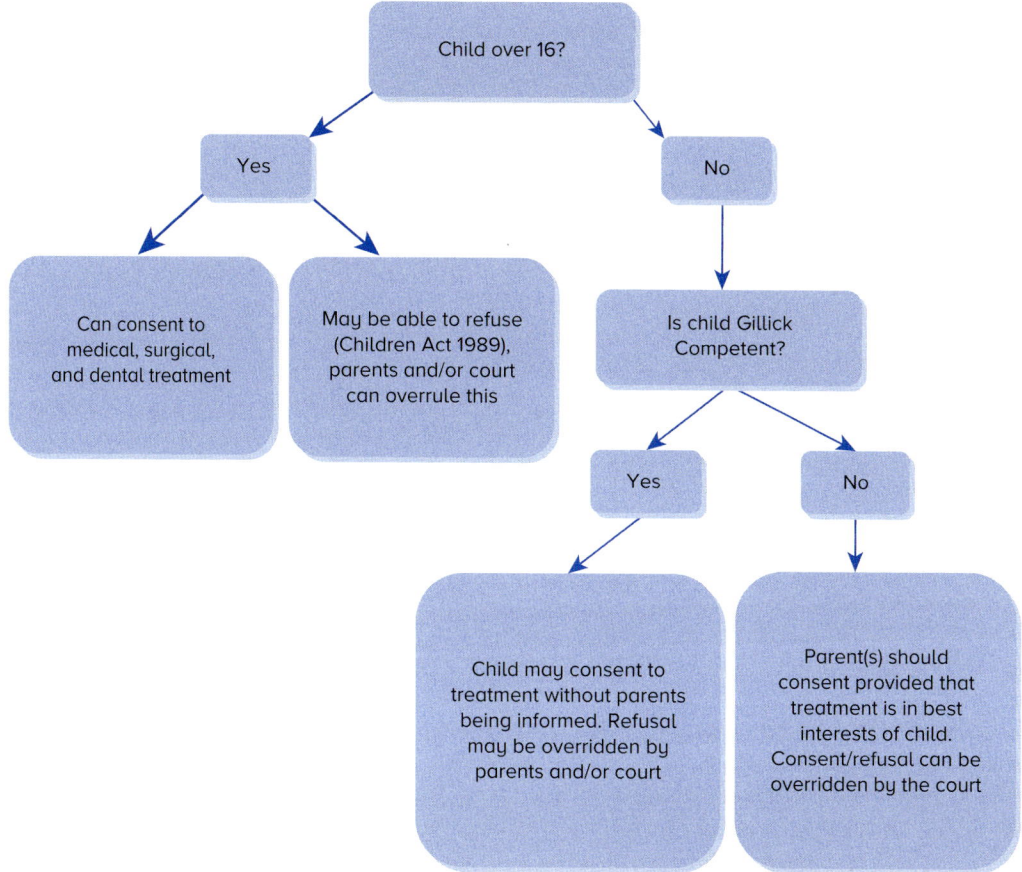

Figure 14.1 Flowchart for determining capacity to consent in children.

Source: adapted from Avery (2017)

Considerations of the responsibilities of parents

The Children Act 1989 defines parental responsibility as 'all the rights, duties and powers, responsibilities and authority which by law a parent has in relation to a child and [their] property' (Section 3(1)). Some of these rights include choosing education, providing a home and naming the child. For healthcare, there is the statutory right for parents to apply for access to medical records and the right to consent or refuse medical treatment on their behalf. However, as noted above, the competence of the child can affect this right. As a child gains competence, they gain the right to be included in decision making and in making decisions about themselves. At the age of 18 (16 in Scotland), parental responsibility for the child ceases. Up to this point, then, the responsibilities of the parent(s) and the rights of the child to be autonomous must be balanced, and as the child gains competence and maturity, the reduction of parental responsibility is reflected accordingly (Cornock, 2011).

Adverse childhood experiences

The conditions that surround a child or young person can greatly affect their health and wellbeing not just during childhood, but across their lifespan. Stressful events during childhood, typically known as adverse childhood experiences can include:

- Domestic violence
- Parental abandonment
- A parent with a mental health condition or chronic illness
- Experiencing abuse – physical, sexual, emotional
- Experiencing neglect – physical, emotional
- Having a household member in prison
- Parental substance misuse.

Adverse childhood experiences are associated with a range of health and social problems during the life-course including mental and physical ill health, suicide, homelessness, drug and alcohol use and criminality (Lewer et al., 2020). Although focus has often been on the longer-term effects of trauma in childhood, Nelson et al. (2020) describe the impact of malnutrition, maltreatment, witnessing violence and experiencing poverty in the first three years of life as ones which can adversely change the developmental trajectory of the child. Because children rely and depend on caregivers for protection and their survival, trauma can greatly impact their ability to make or maintain relationships with others. They may display behaviours which are odd, unusual or concerning (Kirkbride, 2018), thus making it difficult for clinicians to understand or interpret what is happening to a child. Children who have experienced traumas such as abuse are less likely to have developed the resources or resilience to be able to cope and may easily be overwhelmed by their experiences, seeking maladaptive coping strategies such as self-harm.

Although adverse childhood experiences can occur across all populations, it is recognised that these are more likely to occur where a child is living in higher areas of deprivation and poverty. That is not to say that attention should not be paid to the situation of a young person where there is obvious material wealth; clinicians need to be attentive to any sign of abuse or neglect.

Developmental perspectives

Child development, which often involves theories of social, emotional and physical development, is thought to be affected by the surroundings of the child and the caregivers. Grounded in humanistic ideas, John Bowlby's theory of attachment (1969) centred on the need for the child to have a warm, intimate and continuous relationship with a caregiver in which satisfaction and enjoyment are experienced; a child may then develop their sense of self, acceptance and how reliable the people in the world around them are at meeting their emotional and physical needs. Where a child is not securely attached, they may be at risk of not understanding emotional states, whether their own or others, and how to self-regulate their emotions. Where traumas within relationships have occurred, the child may have great difficulty in forming trusting relationships with adults during childhood and adult life.

Adolescence brings about changes to key areas for development: physiological, cognitive, social, emotional and sexual. Puberty is often used as the biological marker for the start of adolescence, around 10 years for girls and 12 for boys, and is thought to end in the late teens. Adolescence can be characterised by significant physical growth alongside cognitive changes, such as moral development, abstract thinking (for example, problem solving and critical thinking), a focus on the self and thinking about others along with developing a sense of identity as to who they are and where they fit in their world.

Adolescence can be a time for experimentation; this allows a young person to try behaviours, gauge other people's responses and learn about themselves. As young people mature through adolescence they can achieve less dependence and oversight from parents, which allows freedoms to explore and experiment. Influences and challenges to this can be felt from parents and peers and they may engage in risk-taking behaviours such as drug and alcohol use, antisocial behaviours and sexual behaviour. Although these are normative aspects to this developmental period they can be problematic where a young person has experienced traumas and adverse childhood experiences. Where there are challenges to development as a result of mental health problems or other long-term conditions, successfully navigating these aspects of adolescence can be more difficult, and there is a possibility of difficulty in adapting and working through these developmental tasks.

Common mental health conditions in children and young people

Emotional disorders

Emotional disorders include anxiety disorders, depressive disorders and mania and bipolar disorders. Roughly one in twelve 5- to 19-year-olds have an emotional disorder (NHS Digital, 2018), which is thought be an increasing trend and is the most common type of disorder experienced by young people. Depression is typified by low mood and a loss of interest in normally enjoyable activities. Lack of energy, anger, guilt, hopelessness, irritability and poor concentration are just some of the emotions or feelings that can also characterise depression. For young people the depression may be influenced by factors around them such as loss of significant family, friends, parental separation, moving house and being away from friends, bullying, abuse and other adverse events. The development of online social media platforms has appeared to influence children's mental health, presenting even more challenges to navigate. Children with a mental disorder were found to use social media on a more frequent basis, for longer, and were more likely to compare themselves to others and be affected by the number of 'likes' they received than those without (NHS Digital, 2018). Young people with a mental disorder are also around twice as likely to be bullied and twice as likely to be cyberbullied than other children. Adolescents who experience cyberbullying are also at increased risk for developing a range of mental health problems, reporting feelings of fear, anxiety and depression (Hoge, Bickham and Cantor, 2017).

Somatic symptoms, that is, medically unexplained physical symptoms such as stomach ache or headaches can be a frequent occurrence where young people have a depressive disorder. Younger children may complain about physical symptoms such as stomach ache more than adolescents and headaches are often associated with depressive disorder. Clinicians should be mindful of unexplained physical symptoms as these can indicate anxiety or depression in young people (Masi et al., 2000; Halayem et al., 2014).

Self-harm and suicide

Children and young people who have a mental disorder are more likely to self-harm. Self-harm is a complex, sensitive and increasingly common occurrence in children and young people. As a way of coping, self-harm can provide short-term relief from difficult feelings. However, it is associated with an increased risk of suicide, increased reliance and addictive behaviours towards self-harm, and unhelpful negative emotions and feelings after self-harming. Self-harm is not a mental disorder as such, but it can strongly indicate underlying problems. Some of the reasons a young person might self-harm are as follows (Mind 2020):

- To express something that is hard to put into words
- To turn invisible thoughts or feelings into something visible
- To change emotional pain into physical pain
- To reduce overwhelming emotional feelings or thoughts
- To gain a sense of being in control
- To escape traumatic memories
- To have something in life that they can rely on
- To punish themselves for their feelings and experiences

- To stop feeling numb, disconnected or dissociated

- In order to create a reason to physically care for themselves

- To express suicidal feelings and thoughts without taking their own life.

When assessing a child who has self-harmed it is important to include the following:

- Any safeguarding concerns, e.g. abuse – physical, emotional, sexual, relating to the child and also to any siblings

- Neglect by caregivers

- Family stressors, e.g. parental separation or divorce

- Internet/social media interfaces, e.g. cyber bullying, web communities

- Bullying by peers

- History of peers who have died by suicide; this may cause trauma and guilt which increases risk

- Previous suicide attempts and if help was sought and how it was sought.

Further information on self-harm can be found in Chapter 10 – Self-harm (p. 127).

Hyperactivity disorders

These disorders are characterised by three aspects: inattention, impulsivity and hyperactivity. Around 1 in 60 children aged 5 to 19 have a hyperactivity disorder in England (NHS Digital, 2018), and there is a higher rate in boys, around four times more, than in girls. Treatment for ADHD (Attention Deficit Hyperactivity Disorder) is typically a combination of psychological, educational and pharmacological treatments. Medication is used to treat the symptoms of ADHD, hyperactivity and impulsivity and also to improve concentration. The most common medications are stimulants such as methylphenidate, amphetamine and dextroamphetamine and non-stimulants such as atomoxetine. This latter medication is used where side effects from stimulants have not been tolerated or where the young person has not wanted to use a stimulant. Usual side effects from these medications include loss of appetite, sleep disturbance, headache and stomach ache so clinicians should be mindful when assessing a young person who is describing these symptoms and is being treated for ADHD. These side effects tend to be short lasting and occur when newly started on these medications.

Autism Spectrum Disorders (ASD)

These disorders affect around 1% of children and young people. It is often found that children with ASD will have difficulty with social interactions and can often misread or interpret the meaning of something differently (Padmore, 2016). For instance, asking a teenager if they have 'had a drink tonight', implying an alcoholic drink, may be interpreted more literally as just a 'drink' so would reply 'yes'. Without clarification this could mislead the clinician into thinking that the young person had consumed alcohol. The same applies if the young person is asked about 'drugs' if they had taken paracetamol for example. This is also indicative of the rigid thinking and impairment to imagination that may be present. As such, communication with a child who has a diagnosis of ASD must be carefully considered and adapted to their needs. Guidance from parents, and from the child, will be invaluable and care and sensitivity in the language used with a child is imperative. Disruptions to routine can be hard for a child with ASD and they may find it difficult in new surroundings with lots of stimulus. They may need to use familiar safety behaviours or use familiar objects to help them focus. Speaking to parents about this is therefore important if conveying a child to hospital.

Assessing and managing children within an ambulance setting

Engaging the child and young person is often the key element to forming a relationship with them. Most children will sense when they are being patronised and will tell you so directly! It is often best to be transparent and speak in terms that are plain and understandable while including the child as much as possible. Careful use of language that both explains what is happening and what you would like to do and involving them in decision making (even if they are not able to consent) are important. Dismissing the child or talking solely with the parent/carer is best avoided so that the young person feels part of the process. Use of exploring questions, such as what, why, when and how will provide an opportunity for a child to explain in their terms what has happened or how they are feeling. Importantly, this may be the first time they have spoken to a healthcare professional about their mental health situation, how they are feeling or their life experiences. It is therefore paramount that these are acknowledged and given time and recognition. A young person may feel ashamed or embarrassed by how they feel or with events that required them to have pre-hospital care; it is vital that this is also recognised and not dismissed as unimportant or left unacknowledged. Having feelings validated will allow a child to see that their problems are being taken seriously and professionally by services. Children and young people, like most people, tend to respond well to humour and honesty, but it is important to be mindful of the type of humour used so it does not make the young person's feelings worse, for example, embarrassment. Engaging can often mean thinking creatively, for example, using observational skills to prompt conversation while assessing a child in their bedroom or taking an interest in their activities or hobbies.

Assessing a child or young person requires mindful attention to the legal requirements previously discussed alongside risk, physical health, mental health, social and environmental factors. Mindful attention may be challenging for clinicians to perform in a very short space of time. While not exhaustive, considering these aspects will help inform the professionals who may see the child next. There is a professional responsibility to report any safeguarding concerns and refer as per local policy and protocol. Reporting risk is also of importance, as is the consideration of risks (which may also align with signs of abuse) from others, such as bullying, violence, domestic violence and abuse, asylum-seeking, racism, as well as risk to self, such as through self-harm, self-poisoning and attempts at suicide.

You may be involved in helping to convey a young person with mental health needs to a mental health hospital. There is no lower age limit within the Mental Health Act (1983[2007]), and it can be used to detain a child for assessment and/or treatment of their mental disorder. A person under the age of 16 and who is not Gillick competent or who is refusing treatment may have consent given by the person or persons who have parental responsibility for the child.

Support for children (signposting)

It will be helpful to be familiar with the referral processes in the local area. Child and Adolescent Mental Health Services (CAMHS) often have a single point of access where referrals can be made by anyone, so offering this advice to the child, parents or carers can be useful.

Helpful information for clinicians and/or carers

- NICE Guideline [NG134] – Depression in children and young people: identification and management at https://www.nice.org.uk/guidance/ng134

- NICE Guideline [NG128] – Autism spectrum disorder in under 19s: recognition, referral and diagnosis at https://www.nice.org.uk/guidance/cg128

- NICE Clinical knowledge summary – Management of self-harm at https://cks.nice.org.uk/topics/self-harm/

- Self-harm in young people: for parents and carers – Royal College of Psychiatrists at https://www.rcpsych.ac.uk/mental-health/parents-and-young-people/information-for-parents-and-carers/self-harm-in-young-people-for-parents-and-carers

- Self-harm: https://www.rcpsych.ac.uk/mental-health/problems-disorders/self-harm

- Non-suicidal self-injury: MHFA Guidelines (Australia) at https://mhfa.com.au/sites/default/files/nssi_mhfa_guidelines_2020_0.pdf; Suicidal thoughts and behaviours: MHFa Guidelines at https://mhfa.com.au/sites/default/files/suicidal_thoughts_and_behaviours_-_mhfa_guidelines_2020_0.pdf

- ADHD Foundation at https://www.adhdfoundation.org.uk/

Support for young people

- Selfharm (www.selfharm.co.uk) – provides support for young people affected by self-harm and has online support groups.

- YoungMinds (www.youngminds.org.uk) – for leaflets written for children about self-harm.

- Harmless (www.harmless.org.uk) – provides support and information to people who self-harm, their friends and families; training for healthcare professionals.

- Mind (www.mind.org.uk) – provides information and support, helplines, local support groups and publications aimed at anyone who self-harms and their friends and family.

- National Self Harm Network (www.nshn.co.uk) – aims to support, empower, and educate people who self-harm and their families and carers.

- Rethink Mental Illness (www.rethink.org) – provides a comprehensive factsheet about self-harm.

- Royal College of Psychiatrists (www.rcpsych.ac.uk) – provides a variety of factsheets.

- Sane (www.sane.org.uk) – campaigns to raise mental health awareness and provides emotional support, practical help, and information including online support.

- The Samaritans (www.samaritans.org) – provides a 24-hour confidential telephone helpline for anyone in a crisis: 08457 909090.

References

Avery G. (2017). *Law and Ethics in Nursing and Healthcare*, 2nd edition. London: Sage.

Clements C. et al. (2016). Rates of self-harm presenting to general hospitals: A comparison of data from the Multicentre Study of Self-Harm in England and Hospital Episode Statistics. *BMJ Open*, 6(2): e009749.

Cornock M. (2011). Parental rights and responsibilities in law. *Nursing Children and Young People*, 23(9): 23–24.

Cornock M. (2015). The child and consent. *Orthopaedic & Trauma Times*, 27: 13–15.

Erskine H. et al. (2015). A heavy burden on young minds: the global burden of mental and substance use disorders in children and youth. *Psychological Medicine*, 45(7): 1551–1563.

Gadancheva V., Barry H. and McNicholas F. (2019). Adolescents Presenting with Mental Health Crises. *Irish Medical Journal*, 112(10): P1020.

Halayem S. et al. (2014). Manifestations d'allure somatique chez l'enfant déprimé: le cas des plaintes somatiques et des conversions [Somatic manifestations among depressed children: the case of complains and conversion symptoms]. *Tunisie Medicale*, 92(2): 154–158.

Hawton K. et al. (2015). Interventions for self-harm in children and adolescents. *Cochrane Database of Systematic Reviews*, 12: CD012013.

HM Government (2018). Working Together to Safeguard Children: A guide to inter-agency working to safeguard and promote the welfare of children. Available at: https://assets.publishing.service.gov.uk/government/uploads/system/uploads/attachment_data/file/942454/Working_together_to_safeguard_children_inter_agency_guidance.pdf

Hoge E., Bickham D. and Cantor J. (2017). Digital Media, Anxiety, and Depression in Children. *Pediatrics*, 140(s2): 76–80.

Jones P. (2013). Adult mental health disorders and their age at onset. *British Journal of Psychiatry*, 202(54): 5–10.

Joseph E. (2018). Fourfold increase in ambulance call outs to children in mental health crisis. Available at: https://www.bournemouthecho.co.uk/news/17230467.fourfold-increase-ambulance-call-outs-children-mental-health-crisis/

Kessler R.C., Amminger G.P. and Aguilar-Gaxiola S. (2007). Age of onset of mental disorders: A review of recent literature. *Current Opinion in Psychiatry*, 20(4): 359–64.

Kirkbride R. (2018). *Counselling Young People*. London: Sage.

Lewer D. et al. (2020). The ACE Index: mapping childhood adversity in England. *Journal of Public Health*, 42(4): e487–e495.

MacDonald K., Fainman-Adelman N., Anderson K.K. and Iyer S.N. (2018). Pathways to mental health services for young people: a systematic review. *Social Psychiatry and Psychiatric Epidemiology*, 53(10): 1005–1038.

McGorry P. (2017). Youth mental health and mental wealth: reaping the rewards. *Australasian Psychiatry*, 25(2): 101–103.

Masi G. et al. (2000). Somatic symptoms in children and adolescents referred for emotional and behavioral disorders. *Psychiatry*, 63(2): 140–149.

Mind (2020). Self-harm. Available at: https://www.mind.org.uk/information-support/types-of-mental-health-problems/self-harm/about-self-harm/

NHS Digital (2018). Mental Health of Children and Young People in England, 2017 Summary of key findings. Available at: https://files.digital.nhs.uk/A6/EA7D58/MHCYP%202017%20Summary.pdf

NHS Digital (2020). Mental Health of Children and Young People in England, 2020: Wave 1 follow up to the 2017 survey. Available at: https://digital.nhs.uk/data-and-information/publications/statistical/mental-health-of-children-and-young-people-in-england/2020-wave-1-follow-up

ONS (2015). Deaths registered in England and Wales (series DR): 2015. Available at: https://www.ons.gov.uk/peoplepopulationandcommunity/birthsdeathsandmarriages/deaths/bulletins/deathsregisteredinenglandandwalesseriesdr/2015

ONS (2020). Leading causes of death, UK: 2001 to 2018. Available at: https://www.ons.gov.uk/peoplepopulationandcommunity/healthandsocialcare/causesofdeath/articles/leadingcausesofdeathuk/2001to2018

Owens D., Horrocks J. and House A. (2002). Fatal and non-fatal repetition of self-harm: Systematic review. *British Journal of Psychiatry*, 181: 193–199.

Padmore J. (2015). *The Mental Health Needs of Children and Young People*. Open University Press: Maidenhead.

Polanczyk G.V. et al. (2015). Annual research review: a meta-analysis of the worldwide prevalence of mental disorders in children and adolescents. *Journal of Child Psychology and Psychiatry*, 56(3): 345–365.

Radez J. et al. (2021). Why do children and adolescents (not) seek and access professional help for their mental health problems? A systematic review of quantitative and qualitative studies. *European Child and Adolescent Psychiatry*, 30: 183–211.

Royal College of Paediatrics and Child Health (2019). Time to raise the standard: children presenting to emergency departments in mental health crisis. Available at: https://www.rcpch.ac.uk/news-events/news/time-raise-standard-children-presenting-emergency-departments-mental-health-crisis

Sadler K. et al. (2018). Mental Health of Children and Young People in England, 2017: Trends and characteristics. Available at: https://openaccess.city.ac.uk/id/eprint/23650/

Turner C. (2021). More children admitted to hospital for mental health than medical reasons, leading paediatrician says. Available at: https://www.telegraph.co.uk/news/2021/01/19/children-admitted-hospital-mental-health-medical-reasons-leading/

Wadman R. et al. (2020). 'These Things Don't Work.' Young People's Views on Harm Minimization Strategies as a Proxy for Self-Harm: A Mixed Methods Approach. *Archives of Suicide Research*, 24(3): 384–401.

World Health Organization (2014). Health for the world's adolescents: a second chance in the second decade. Available at: https://www.who.int/publications/i/item/WHO-FWC-MCA-14.05

World Health Organization (2020). Adolescent mental health. Available at: https://www.who.int/news-room/fact-sheets/detail/adolescent-mental-health

Young S. (2018). A&E attendances by young people with mental health problems havealmost doubled in five years. *The Independent* Available at: https://www.independent.co.uk/life-style/mental-health-young-people-and-e-department-health-and-social-care-figures-a8600596.html

Drugs and Alcohol and the Impact on Mental Health Response

Chapter 15

David Partlow

Understanding substance use

First, it is very important to acknowledge that recreational drug use and alcohol are not issues relevant only to mental health, nor should they be considered mental health issues per se. We do, however, need to acknowledge the relationship that is often seen between the use of such substances and mental health crisis.

The use of recreational drugs and alcohol has long been an issue in an emergency context, many paramedics will recall their experiences attempting to engage mental health services for patients who are intoxicated or otherwise incapacitated.

For some though, the use of substances is far more complex. Harris and Edlund (2005) conclude that substance use was consistent with the suggestion that self-medication was a significant factor and, further, that earlier intervention to reduce unmet need could reduce the development of substance use disorders. If self-medication is a factor, immediate withdrawal can in certain cases be problematic and negatively impact on the wellbeing of the individual. We should not, therefore, consider substance use in a wholly negative context and while this may be a factor in the developing mental health need, it may also provide an individual with an element of control. As such, the balance between mental health needs and substance use needs is a complex presentation that cannot be resolved quickly.

Self-medicating may take a number of forms, including consumption of alcohol and recreational drug use, but may also involve prescription drugs and nicotine (smoking). An interesting question to ask, although unrelated to the major topic here, is the use of food as a self-medicating strategy and links to the complex issue of the inter-relationship between physical and mental health and the social determinants of health.

The World Health Organization (WHO, 2014) highlights risk factors that exist for mental health disorders and associated links with social inequality. Inadequate housing, poor education and poverty are closely associated with exposure to alcohol addiction and drug misuse and thus to poor health outcomes and higher mortality. What is difficult to quantify is whether social inequality leads to behaviours that are of themselves risk factors for poor mental health or whether, in some cases, the reverse is true and that poor mental health leads to behaviours that create a risk of poor physical health. What is likely is that both are true and that we cannot separate a conversation about physical health from a conversation about mental health, as both are fundamental components of each other.

Self-medication is often evident when the use of alcohol or drugs is triggered by anxiety or mental anguish. In such cases it is possible that drugs and alcohol temporarily alleviate the pain, but, as long-term resolution cannot be achieved, the drug and alcohol use may increase as tolerance builds and increasing amounts are required to gain effect. The downward spiral that can develop can lead to deterioration in a host of physical problems, all of which can increase sources of tension and anxiety, further increasing the impact on mental health of the individual. Significant physical health issues include liver disease, high blood pressure, development of certain cancers and a range of mental health problems including depression, anxiety and episodes of drug-induced psychosis (Rethink Mental Illness, 2020).

Alcohol

Alcohol is freely available and in certain contexts its use is encouraged and the societal norm. The Mental Health Foundation (2006) described it as 'the UKs favourite coping mechanism'.

The association with poor health outcomes is well known; the Scottish Government in introducing minimum unit pricing (MUP) suggested in 2016 that they would see 400 fewer alcohol-related deaths within five years and manage 8,000 fewer alcohol-related hospital admissions. Anderson et al. (2019) reviewed the immediate impact and concluded that alcohol sales had reduced in Scottish households, although further work was required to look at this strategy over the longer term to determine if these outcomes had been delivered. Data did show that there were 116 fewer alcohol-specific deaths in Scotland in 2019 compared to 2018 (National Records of Scotland, 2021).

It is estimated that there are 589,000 individuals resident in England who live with alcohol dependency (O'Connor, 2020). Of those, around 147,000 are likely to be in receipt of medication for anxiety and depression, among other mental health disorders. Alcohol used in moderation can be associated with improved mood and emotional wellbeing, but taken in excess it can lead to significant issues related to both physical and mental ill-health.

Data from The Mental Health Foundation (2006) suggests that as many as 65% of suicides have a link to excessive drinking and 70% of men who die by suicide have consumed alcohol prior to taking their own lives. This is supported by a report from Public Health England (2016) which stated that a review of the relationship between addiction and suicide reported that between 10% and 69% of completed suicides tested positive for alcohol use and 10% to 73% of attempted suicides tested positive for alcohol use.

We know that drinking too much alcohol causes damage to the nerve cells within the brain, we also know that regular alcohol intake can cause damage to blood vessels in the brain and disrupt the provision of thiamine (vitamin B1) and serotonin. So, the physical impact on neurological functioning is clear. There are, though, other associated factors such as increased propensity to poor self-care, increased likelihood of self-neglect and other damaging activities such as smoking and poor dietary choice and a greater potential for negative socioeconomic impact. This therefore creates a developing negative cycle where alcohol and poor mental health are intrinsically linked, each sustaining and developing the other.

Whether alcohol intake is responsible for mental ill-health or whether poor mental health leads to increased alcohol intake as a coping mechanism is unique to individual circumstances, but what is important for paramedic practice is that the individual in need of care and support is able to access treatment without judgement or preconceived notions based on societal norms.

When conducting an assessment of an individual's needs, it is important to see beyond the current state of intoxication, to consider the individual at the centre and to ensure that every opportunity is taken to break the cycle of disruptive behaviours.

Common illicit substances

Categorisation of illicit substances provides a level of understanding relating to the potential impact.

Cannabinoids

These include cannabis and marijuana; they are generally smoked or swallowed in order to create a sense of euphoria or relaxation. Cannabis use can provide a period of relaxation and a removal of inhibitions similar to alcohol. It can however also create a degree of lethargy, and in some cases mild hallucinations, anxiety and paranoia. Symptoms associated with drug-induced psychosis may increase if cannabis is used frequently or for a prolonged period of time. The Royal College of Psychiatrists (2015) suggests that individuals who are perhaps more likely to develop mental health problems, through familial history for example, face increased risks of early development of mental ill-health if they use cannabis regularly.

Cannabis can also become addictive, particularly if the individual has started using it in early life and over a prolonged period. Individuals may also develop a tolerance such that the amount required to produce the same effect increases. This, in turn, can lead to withdrawal symptoms including irritability, cravings, restlessness and problems sleeping.

Street names include:
- Cannabis: bhang, bud, doob, dope, ganja, grass, hash, hashish, Mary-Jane, pot, skunk, spliff, weed.

Opioids

These are generally injected, smoked, swallowed or snorted to create a sense of euphoria. Heroin can enable the user to feel relaxed as it can generate a feeling of calm, but it carries a significant risk when taken with other substances including alcohol, potentially leading to overdose. Heroin is particularly addictive and can have significant long-term effects, which can be compounded by methods of administration and serious risk of infection.

Street names include:

- Heroin: brown, gear, H, horse, junk, skag, smack.

Stimulants

Stimulants are generally snorted, smoked, injected and swallowed. They often create significant risk of tachycardias, hypertension and pyrexia. Cocaine can increase confidence and stimulate the individual; it can also be addictive and can lead to cocaine toxicity, cardiac arrythmias and death. Cocaine can also create an imbalance in dopamine in the brain and thereby cause or exacerbate pre-existing depression and schizophrenia.

Amphetamine and methamphetamine are taken to increase the level of alertness. These drugs can subsequently create difficulties with sleep and the ability to relax. They can be addictive and again, lead to drug-induced psychosis anxiety and depression.

Street names include:

- Amphetamine: base, billy, paste, speed, sulph, whizz.
- Cocaine: blow, Chang, Ching, Charlie, coke, flake, sniff, snow, white.
- Methamphetamine: crank, crystal meth, glass, ice, meth.

Club drugs

Club drugs are an increasingly common illicit substance; they can be swallowed, snorted or injected with a variety of effects depending on the substance itself. Some of the drugs in this category have been previously described as 'legal highs'. Until a change in the law in 2016, many such substances were legally available.

The term 'New Psychoactive Substance' is used to describe a myriad of drugs and includes stimulants, sedatives, hallucinogens and synthetic cannabinoids, the most common of which is known as spice. The short- and longer-term effects vary widely, but many can be extremely dangerous, particularly when used alongside alcohol or other sedatives.

The Royal Society of Psychiatrists (2015) identified that individuals who used new psychoactive substances often experienced mental health problems and were at an increased risk of developing a psychological dependency.

Street names include:

- New psychoactive substances: bath salts, Dimethocaine, Eric 3, Mdat, Nps, Plant Food.

- Synthetic cannabinoids: Amsterdam gold, black mamba, clockwork orange, spice.

Dissociative drugs

These illicit substances can be chewed, smoked, injected, snorted and swallowed depending on the substance. They create a variety of effects but as a group are considered to generate a feeling of separation, of being outside or dissociated from the body.

Ketamine produces a detached state which can create an altered perception of time and space. There are a number of physical health risks associated with long-term use, including: tachycardias, significant bladder, urinary tract and kidney problems, alongside liver damage and abdominal pain. Ketamine can also cause depression and may also create additional psychotic symptoms including hallucinations. Ketamine can also exacerbate any pre-existing mental health conditions. Those individuals who use ketamine regularly can also develop a tolerance to it, leading to increased dosage and subsequent risk of significant side effects and potentially death. Ketamine withdrawal does not produce physical symptoms and therefore the addiction is considered to be a psychological dependence.

De Gregorio (2021) outlines the emergence of a number of clinical studies that are reviewing the potential of hallucinogens in the treatment of psychiatric disorders. Multiple clinical studies have reviewed the potential benefits of ketamine in the treatment of depressive disorders and further evidence is currently being evaluated looking at the potential use of other substances, such as LSD and MDMA, in the treatment of post-traumatic stress disorders.

Street names include:

- Ketamine: donkey dust, green, K, ket, Kit Kat, Special K, super K, vitamin K, wonk.

Hallucinogens

Hallucinogens are commonly swallowed, smoked, and absorbed through mucosal membranes. These include naturally occurring hallucinogens such as psilocybin mushrooms and peyote cactus (mescaline). In addition, hallucinogens may be chemically synthesised, such as phencyclidine (commonly known as PCP or angel dust), lysergic acid diethylamide (LSD), and 3,4-Methylenedioxymethamphetamine, or MDMA (commonly known as ecstasy).

Similar to cocaine, ecstasy can create a feeling of positive energy, but can also lead to significant anxiety and produce drug-induced psychosis. Hallucinogens can also create panic attacks, increased risk of violent behaviours, agitation, paranoia, depression, and terror.

The use of hallucinogens can cause long-term psychosis leading to visual disturbances, flashbacks, paranoia and anxiety. Hallucinogen use can lead to a significant deterioration in an individual's mental health, and also significantly impact on an individual's pre-existing mental ill-health.

Street names include:

- LSD: acid, blotter, dots, L, liquid acid, micro dot, tabs, trippers, window.
- MDMA: E, ecstasy, MD, Mandy, Molly, pills.
- PCP: angel dust, hog, peace pills.
- Psilocybin mushrooms: liberty caps, mushies, shrooms.

Drug interactions

While it is not always possible to predict or describe the potential symptoms caused by the interaction between prescribed medication and illicit substances, the combination increases the risk of adverse effects and should always be noted when conducting an assessment of an individual where this is a consideration.

Mind (2016) outlines a number of known effects and highlights the increased risk that occurs with multiple interactions. These include potentially fatal interactions such as the use of heroin and benzodiazepines where the depressant effect is enhanced leading to respiratory or cardiac arrest. Concordant use of citalopram (an SSRI antidepressant) with cocaine, significantly increases the risk of haemorrhage and hypertension.

References

Anderson P. et al. (2019). Impact of minimum unit pricing on alcohol purchases in Scotland and Wales: controlled interrupted time series analysis. *The Lancet*, 6(8): E557–E565.

Cornah D. and the Mental Health Foundation (2006). Cheers? Understanding the relationship between alcohol and mental health. Available at: https://www.drugsandalcohol.ie/15771/1/cheers_report%5B1%5D.pdf

De Gregorio D. et al. (2021). Hallucinogens in Mental Health: Preclinical and Clinical Studies on LSD, Psilocybin, MDMA, and Ketamine. *Journal of Neuroscience*, 41(5): 891–900.

Harris K. and Edlund M. (2005). Self-Medication of Mental Health Problems: New Evidence from a National Survey. *Health Services Research*, 40(1): 117–134.

Mental Health Foundation (2006). Cheers? Understanding the relationship between alcohol and mental health. Available at: https://www.mentalhealth.org.uk/sites/default/files/cheers_report.pdf

Mind (2016). Recreational drugs and alcohol. Available at: https://www.Mind.org.uk/information-support/types-of-mental-health-problems/drugs-recreational-drugs-alcohol/recreational-drugs-medication/

National Records of Scotland (2021). Alcohol specific deaths. Available at: https://www.nrscotland.gov.uk/statistics-and-data/statistics/statistics-by-theme/vital-events/deaths/alcohol-deaths

NHS (2021). Cannabis: the facts. Healthy body. Available at: https://www.nhs.uk/live-well/healthy-body/cannabis-the-facts/

O'Connor R. (2020). Alcohol dependence and mental health. Available at: https://publichealthmatters.blog.gov.uk/2020/11/17/alcohol-dependence-and-mental-health/

Public Health England (2016). The Public Health Burden of Alcohol and the Effectiveness and Cost-Effectiveness of Alcohol Control Policies: An evidence review. Available at: https://assets.publishing.service.gov.uk/government/uploads/system/uploads/attachment_data/file/733108/alcohol_public_health_burden_evidence_review_update_2018.pdf

Rethink Mental Illness (2020). Drugs, alcohol and mental health. Available at: https://www.rethink.org/advice-and-information/about-mental-illness/learn-more-about-conditions/drugs-alcohol-and-mental-health/

Royal College of Psychiatrists (2015). Cannabis and mental health: for young people. Available at: https://www.rcpsych.ac.uk/mental-health/parents-and-young-people/young-people/cannabis-and-mental-health-information-for-young-people

Royal College of Psychiatrists (2015). Club Drugs. Available at: https://www.rcpsych.ac.uk/mental-health/parents-and-young-people/young-people/club-drugs?searchTerms=new%20psychoactive%20substances

World Health Organization (WHO, 2014). Social determinants of mental health. Available at: https://www.who.int/publications/i/item/9789241506809

Conclusion

We have all experienced a number of difficulties in our lives – while this book has been in production, we have experienced a global pandemic that has created a range of challenges, both personal and professional that we have all had to overcome. It is, therefore, important that when reading this book, we don't consider ourselves immune to the mental health challenges that come with working as paramedics and that we take the opportunity to reflect on how we cope with increased stress and what mechanisms we can employ to stay well.

While the paramedic profession is challenging, it is important that we don't engage in conversations that are totally negative. Some of us will have found life during the COVID-19 pandemic incredibly restrictive and difficult and found that this has impacted on our mental wellbeing, but others will have found opportunities for personal growth and have discovered just what they can achieve when times get hard.

Remember!

It is OK to not be OK, but equally it's OK to be OK when challenges come thick and fast. We are all individuals and as we also respond to physical challenges in different ways, so we respond to mental challenges in an equal array of ways. That's what makes each one of us unique and that's what makes our responses unique to us.

We hope that through this book we have been able to provide some insight into mental health conditions and the challenges that can be presented to paramedics on a professional level. All those who work in challenging professions should take time to consider their own mental wellbeing.

In aspects of good physical health, prevention strategies are key, and so it is with mental health. So consider your coping mechanisms, recognise what you do to stay well and invest time and energy in developing healthy practices. Whether this is through human connection, through continued learning and education, through the act of giving to others, combined with healthy eating and exercise, or through other pursuits or social activities. The work of an operational paramedic can be tough, but it can be highly rewarding and fulfilling. Take time to enjoy the positive while reflecting and managing the impact of the negative.

As a nation we are more aware of the need to think about, and importantly, to talk about mental health. We have all made huge strides in taking this conversation forward. There can be no health without mental health and we are at last waking up to the importance of having those discussions. Mental health is a core component of the ambulance service response. People in crisis have a right to be treated with dignity and respect and in parity with those who have need of support through physical ill-health or incapacity.

The Government White Paper on the reform of the Mental Health Act has also been published and will hopefully bring with it some improvements to the current provision of mental healthcare in this country.

The White Paper (DHSC, 2021) brings with it an end to the use of police cells for the detention of individuals under the Mental Health Act. The provision of the Crisis Care Concordat in 2014 promised a new era where mental health would have equal footing with physical health, a new parity of esteem was promised and with it some improvements at least in the profile of mental health and the commitment of organisations to work together.

The White Paper seeks to address a long-standing issue with regard to the power to detain or hold an individual within an emergency department. Currently, individuals within an emergency department who are not under arrest or detained by the police, may simply leave and there are multiple examples of where individuals have subsequently gone on to harm themselves or others.

Police colleagues have then been pressurised to play a role in managing complex presentations without any real legal power to act. The White Paper seeks to expand the Section 5 of the Mental Health Act 1983 to emergency departments. The holding powers contained within Section 5 currently allow a doctor, or mental health/learning disabilities practitioner to keep an individual in hospital until a Mental Health Act assessment has been completed. The issue at present is that Section 5 cannot be used in an emergency department because it only applies to inpatients within the hospital and individuals within an emergency department are not, legally, classed as inpatients.

In addition, there is a proposal to replace the nearest relative with a nominated person with an associated increase in powers. At present, the nearest relative acts to safeguard the rights of the individual and must be consulted when detention under the Mental Health Act is being considered.

The White Paper also stresses, as did the Crisis Care Concordat and many other papers since, that the transfer of an individual detained under the Mental Health Act or requiring transfer for assessment or management of mental health crisis remains the responsibility of the ambulance service.

As noted earlier, there is no health without mental health, we cannot absolve ourselves of responsibility to support others in crisis and it should never matter whether that crisis is precipitated by physical or mental health. The role of the paramedic is to provide an immediate response, to assess the needs of individuals and to support them in seeking and receiving help.

We have a long way to go to fully embed the principles of parity of esteem and to fully acknowledge the need to view mental ill-health in the same way that we view physical ill-health, but as paramedics we have a pivotal role to play in addressing this disparity and in driving forward the agenda to ensure that all those in need are supported and provided with the levels of care for which the paramedic profession is rightly proud.

References

Department of Health and Social Care (2021). Reforming the Mental Health Act. Available at: https://assets.publishing.service.gov.uk/government/uploads/system/uploads/attachment_data/file/951741/mental-health-act-reform-print.pdf

Crisis Care Concordat. Available at: https://www.crisiscareconcordat.org.uk/

Index